Ty   es
fo   s

▲®**American Diabetes Association**®
Cure • Care • Commitment®

Associate Director, Consumer Books,
Sherrye Landrum; *Editor,* Gregory L. Guthrie, *Associate Director, Book Production,* Peggy M. Rote; *Composition*, Circle Graphics, Inc.; *Cover Design,* Koncept, Inc.; *Printer,* Worzalla Publishing.

Printed in the United States of America
1 3 5 7 9 10 8 6 4 2

The suggestions and information contained in this publication are generally consistent with the *Clinical Practice Recommendations* and other policies of the American Diabetes Association, but they do not represent the policy or position of the Association or any of its boards or committees. Reasonable steps have been taken to ensure the accuracy of the information presented. However, the American Diabetes Association cannot ensure the safety or efficacy of any product or service described in this publication. Individuals are advised to consult a physician or other appropriate health care professional before undertaking any diet or exercise program or taking any medication referred to in this publication. Professionals must use and apply their own professional judgment, experience, and training and should not rely solely on the information contained in this publication before prescribing any diet, exercise, or medication. The American Diabetes Association—its officers, directors, employees, volunteers, and members—assumes no responsibility or liability for personal or other injury, loss, or damage that may result from the suggestions or information in this publication.

⊚ The paper in this publication meets the requirements of the ANSI Standard Z39.48-1992 (permanence of paper).

ADA titles may be purchased for business or promotional use or for special sales. To purchase this book in large quantities, or for custom editions of this book with your logo, contact Lee Romano Sequeira, Special Sales & Promotions, at the address below, or at LRomano@diabetes.org or 703-299-2046.

American Diabetes Association
1701 North Beauregard Street
Alexandria, Virginia 22311

Library of Congress Cataloging-in-Publication Data

Barrier, Phyllis, 1946–
 Type 2 diabetes for beginners / Phyllis Barrier.
  p. cm.
 Includes index.
 ISBN 1-58040-224-0
 1. Non-insulin-dependent diabetes—Popular works. I. Title: Type two diabetes for beginners. II. Title.

 RC662.18.B37 2005
 616.4'62—dc22

                              2004029175

To the people with diabetes
who have taught me so much
about combining life and diabetes care.

To my parents
and to my husband, Michael.

Contents

Foreword

When we read a book, we read "within the lines" and
"between the lines." "Within the lines" means that
we pay attention to what the author has written, to
the printed facts and the information. "Between the
lines" refers to both the emotional tone in which the
facts and information are given as well as the
information that the author has *not* included.
Type 2 Diabetes for Beginners, which has been
written by a seasoned nutritionist with substantial
diabetes experience, has the comprehensive
information and facts "within" its lines—from carb
counting to stress management—that a person
needs in order to begin and maintain a life with
diabetes. However, what is most unique about this
book is that it also communicates "between the
lines," providing the essential emotional message
that it takes determination, courage, and support
to maintain the stamina to sustain this journey in
living with diabetes. The experienced nutritionist
who wrote *Type 2 Diabetes for Beginners* is also an
experienced clinician and has worked for years with
individuals with diabetes and their families. Phyllis
Barrier understands that what patients and families

need does not simply end at the information and facts, but also requires energy, optimism, and engagement to successfully apply diabetes facts and create and continue healthy lifestyle changes.

As to information that is not included in this book, you will find no mention of how easy it is to live with diabetes. You will not find misleading messages that say you can "do it all yourself." In fact, you are assured that living with diabetes is a difficult challenge and that everyone on the road needs two teams—an experienced health care team and a family/friend support team. What I appreciate most about this book is its honest and reassuring tone. Within the lines and between them, the patient is guided to take small and realistic steps to create and continue needed lifestyle changes. And as Phyllis has said so strongly within and between the lines, building a long and healthy life with diabetes can be a realistic long-term goal for everyone with diabetes.

Barbara Anderson, PhD
Professor, Pediatric Endocrinology and Metabolism
Baylor College of Medicine
Houston, Texas

I am much honored to introduce this book and congratulate you on taking this important step in caring for your diabetes. If you are like many of the people who I see as a diabetes educator and you just found out that you have type 2 diabetes, you are probably feeling somewhat overwhelmed. You may also be feeling angry, scared, or confused.

You probably also have questions. You may have concerns about taking care of a chronic illness such as diabetes. And you may have discovered that diabetes is different from other illnesses you have had. Having diabetes means that there are many decisions to be made each day about how you care for yourself. Making wise choices will make a difference in both how you feel today and your future health.

You may also want to begin to make some changes in your life that will help you take better care of yourself and your diabetes. As much you truly want to make this changes, it is never easy, especially when it comes to how you eat, handle stress, and exercise.

It may help to know that you are not alone. This book is written to be a resource to help you learn how to manage and cope with diabetes. You may not know a lot about diabetes yet, but you do know about yourself and what is important to you. When you combine what you know with what your health care team knows about diabetes, you'll have a powerful combination.

I often tell my patients that diabetes is a journey. It is not probably not a journey that you would have chosen and it is not an easy one. But even the hardest journey is made easier when you can lighten your load. This book can be a guide for you. The more you know, the more you will feel that you are in charge of diabetes, rather than allowing diabetes to control you. You can also learn how to make decisions that are right for you and make changes in your life so that you not only live long but live well.

Best wishes on your journey.

Martha M. Funnell, MS, RN, CDE
Michigan Diabetes Research and Training Center
Ann Arbor, Michigan

Acknowledgments

Len Boswell, Vice President, Publications, American Diabetes Association, came up with the idea for a book that would help people who are just beginning to deal with type 2 diabetes. I am grateful that he asked me to write it.

Many other staff members at the National Office of the American Diabetes Association helped make this book a reality. Special thanks to Sherrye Landrum; John Fedor, Director of Publishing; Abraham Ogden and Gregory Guthrie, Editors; Stephanie Dunbar, MPh, RD, Director of Program Publications; and the illustrators and desktoppers.

Thanks also to the many volunteers I worked with at the American Diabetes Association. They taught me so much through the years. I cannot possibly list them all, but I hope they know who they are! I do want to single out those volunteers who worked with me on the Program Publications Editorial Board: Martha M. Funnell, MS, RN, CDE; Virginia Paragallo-Dittko, MA, RN, CDE; Barbara Anderson, PhD; Patricia Barr, BS; Carol Homko, PhD, RN, CDE; Melinda Maryniuk, MEd, RD, CDE; Catherine Mullooly, MS, CDE; Robin Nwankwo,

MPH, RD, CDE; Cecilia Boyer Casey, MS, RN, CDE; Richard Rubin, PhD, CDE; and Andrea Zaldivar, MS, ANP, CDE. Marion Franz, MS, RD, CDE, and Madelyn Wheeler, MS, RD, were my wonderful nutrition mentors and always had time for a question or volunteer project.

And last, but not least, I want to thank my parents for their sacrifices and support through the years. I also want to thank my husband, Michael, who has been my best friend, sounding board, and "at home editor."

Introduction

Diabetes has been part of my life for many years. You see, diabetes is in my family. My Aunt Carla had diabetes for as long as I can remember. My cousin Pam has diabetes. Now my mom has diabetes. A number of my high school friends now have type 2 diabetes. Many people I love have diabetes. Many people you love probably have type 2 diabetes, too. And you or a family member or friend may have been told you have pre-diabetes or type 2 diabetes.

As a Registered Dietitian (RD), I have worked for more than 25 years with people who have diabetes. I became a Certified Diabetes Educator (CDE) almost 20 years ago. A CDE is a health care provider who specializes in diabetes education. I had to pass a special exam. I have worked in health departments with kids, adults, and pregnant women who had diabetes. I have worked in managed care, helping people learn to take care of their diabetes.

I most recently worked at the National Office for the American Diabetes Association for more than

11 years. I helped write guidelines and booklets for people with type 2 diabetes.

Now the American Diabetes Association has asked me to write this book. The American Diabetes Association has many fine books, but they wanted me to write a book that focuses on the basic stuff— what you really need to know if you've recently been diagnosed with type 2 diabetes. Many people I've worked with through the years have told me, "My life is too busy as it is. Just tell me what I need to do to take care of my diabetes." Well, here it is.

If you've recently been diagnosed with diabetes, you may be scared. You may know about the problems that diabetes has caused in your family or friends. But you may not have heard the good news about having pre-diabetes or type 2 diabetes today:

- You can have a healthy, active, and long life with pre-diabetes or type 2 diabetes.
- You can learn to cope with the ups and downs of living with pre-diabetes or type 2 diabetes.
- You can take care of yourself by using a meal plan, being active most days of the week, and taking diabetes medicines, if needed.
- If you have pre-diabetes, you can delay or prevent getting type 2 diabetes.
- You can delay or prevent long-term problems by caring for your diabetes each day.

When it comes to your diabetes care, the experts agree that you're in charge. Sure, you go to the doctor or see a nurse educator every few months. But you choose what and how much to eat. You decide if you'll take your diabetes medicine, if you'll check your blood sugar, and if you'll be active.

You're in charge, but you're not alone. Lean on your diabetes team for care and support. Who is on your diabetes team? It might be your spouse, your kids, your parents, your friends, or other members of your family. It might be a neighbor you've known for years. It might be people from your church or synagogue or from where you work. Your diabetes health care team can include your doctor, diabetes educator, dietitian, eye doctor, foot doctor, and mental health counselor.

Many of the people on your team may also have diabetes. Today many people in the United States and around the world have diabetes. Eighteen million Americans have diabetes. Forty million more have pre-diabetes. Adults aren't the only ones developing pre-diabetes or type 2 diabetes. Now many kids are also developing pre-diabetes or type 2 diabetes.

There's never a vacation from having diabetes or caring for your diabetes. But as millions of people know, you can live a healthy and happy life with it.

Turn to the table of contents to start learning how. From the list of chapters, you can choose where to start. You may want to zoom to Chapter 7 to learn more about checking blood sugar. Or you may want to start with Chapter 3 and go on to 4, 5, and 6. They deal with food and diabetes. Or you may just want to start at the beginning and read through the book.

Chapter 1

Type 1 and Type 2 Diabetes: What's the Difference?

There are many types of diabetes, but the two most common are type 1 and type 2 diabetes. Diabetes means that your blood sugar, or glucose (GLOO-kos), is too high.

Everyone's blood has some sugar in it because your body needs sugar for energy. Our brain can only work if it has blood sugar. But too much sugar in your blood—too much glucose—can mean you have diabetes. Normally, your body breaks food down into sugar and sends it into your bloodstream. Then your pancreas (PAN-kree-us) makes a hormone called insulin (IN-suh-lin). Insulin's job is to help get the sugar from the blood into your body's cells, where it can be used for energy. Insulin helps keep blood sugar in a normal range.

In type 1 diabetes, the pancreas makes little or no insulin. People with type 1 diabetes get insulin from a shot or a pump to keep their blood sugar in their target range. Most people with type 1 diabetes take two to four shots a day or use an insulin pump. Old names for type 1 diabetes are juvenile-onset diabetes or insulin-dependent diabetes.

People with pre-diabetes or type 2 diabetes still make insulin. But their pancreas may not be making enough or their body may not be using it the right way. People with pre-diabetes or type 2 can manage their diabetes by watching what they eat, by being more active, and sometimes by taking diabetes medicines. Old names for type 2 diabetes are maturity-onset diabetes or adult-onset diabetes, but now kids are getting type 2.

Kids who are overweight and aren't active are more likely to get diabetes. So are kids who have a family member with diabetes. Some racial and ethnic groups have a greater risk of getting diabetes: Native Americans, African Americans, Hispanic Americans (Latinos), Asian Americans, and Pacific Islanders.

Today everyone knows someone who has diabetes. It may be a family member, like your mother, your aunt, or your child. Or it may be a coworker or good friend. When I worked for the American Diabetes Association, I always carried my American Diabetes Association work bag when I traveled on an airplane. Every single time someone on the plane would talk to me about diabetes. They talked about their grandchild's diabetes, about their brother's diabetes, or about their own diabetes.

Diabetes is serious and more people are getting it. By taking care of your diabetes and showing others how to do it, you may prevent people you love from getting diabetes. You can be a role model for people around you.

People with type 1 or type 2 diabetes do some of the same things to care for their diabetes. They watch what they eat, they are active, and they check their blood sugar levels using a meter. But we'll learn more about all of that in later chapters in this book.

Chapter 2

What Is Pre-Diabetes?

Pre-diabetes is a condition that comes before type 2 diabetes. It means that blood sugar levels are higher than normal but aren't high enough to be called diabetes. As we become older, or less active, or gain weight, we are more at risk for pre-diabetes and type 2 diabetes. People can have pre-diabetes and not know it.

If you have pre-diabetes, it means

- you might get type 2 diabetes sometime soon or further down the road.
- you are more likely to get heart disease or have a stroke.

The good news is that you can take steps to delay or prevent type 2 diabetes with

- regular physical activity, such as walking almost every day.
- weight loss.

A recent study, called the Diabetes Prevention Program, showed that these steps helped most people delay or prevent type 2 diabetes. Being active and losing weight worked well for people of all ages.

Being active almost every day is one of the best ways to delay or prevent type 2 diabetes. You can lower your chances of getting type 2 diabetes by adding physical activity to your daily routine. Even if you have heart disease or other problems, you can still be more active. Work with your health care team to find out which physical activities are safe for you.

Along with being more active, weight loss can delay or prevent type 2 diabetes. Reaching a healthy weight can help you a lot. If you're overweight any weight loss, even 5 or 10 pounds, will lower your chances of getting type 2 diabetes.

Losing extra weight helped people in the Diabetes Prevention Program delay or prevent type 2 diabetes. People in the study lost an average of 15 pounds in the first year of the study. How did they do it? They ate fewer calories and less fat. And they exercised most days of the week. In fact, many walked about 150 minutes a week.

It helps to keep track of the progress you're making with eating and walking. Write down everything you eat and drink for a week. Writing things down makes you more aware of what you're eating and helps with weight loss. You can keep track of your walking by wearing a pedometer on your belt. A pedometer is a small device that tells you how many steps you've taken. Or you can keep track of your walking or other activity by writing it down for a week. At the end of the week, total up the minutes you've been active to see how you're doing.

If you have pre-diabetes, you may suspect that someone you love has pre-diabetes or type 2 diabetes. At their next doctor visit, ask them to get their blood sugar checked if they are

- 45 or older.
- under 45 but overweight and at increased risk for diabetes. **Increased risk for diabetes** means they may have one or more of these risk factors:

  - They have a close family member, like a parent, brother, or sister, with diabetes.
  - They are

    - African American
    - Native American
    - Asian American
    - Pacific Islander
    - Hispanic American (Latino)

  - They've had a baby weighing more than nine pounds or they've had gestational diabetes.
  - They have high blood pressure (over 140/90).
  - They have low HDL cholesterol, the good cholesterol (40 or lower).
  - They have high triglycerides (150 or higher).

Small steps lead to big rewards. Taking small steps to change the way you eat and increase your activity can delay or prevent type 2 diabetes. Decide how you'll reduce your calories to lose weight. Think about what you're willing and able to do to be more active almost every day.

Type 2 diabetes is a serious disease. If you delay or prevent it, you'll enjoy better health in the long run. Feeling good and having energy are keys to living the good life.

Chapter 3

Eating and Type 2 Diabetes

When people find out they have type 2 diabetes, the first thing they want to know is what they can eat, when can they eat, and how much they can eat. In fact, studies show that people with diabetes find dealing with food the hardest part of their diabetes care.

Many people think that having diabetes means they can't eat their most favorite foods. But that's just not true. You can still eat the foods you love. By working with your dietitian and by reading this book, you will know how to include your favorite foods and still keep your blood sugar levels on track. For more information on blood sugar goals, see Chapter 8.

For most of us, food means more than just getting full. Eating meals brings us together with family and friends. It brings comfort and pleasure. That's why, for most people with diabetes, food is the toughest part. There's no doubt about it. Changing the way you eat or the times you eat can be really tough. But keep in mind that you're in charge—you can do it.

When you're first told you have diabetes, you may not be able to meet with a dietitian right away. So what do you do? There are many ways to take on diabetes meal planning, so let's talk about some of those ways. The first diabetes meal planning method I'll talk about is called rating your plate.

Rate Your Plate

Life isn't easy, and having diabetes isn't easy. A first step in beginning meal planning is to "rate your plate." With type 2 diabetes, the amount of food you eat affects your blood sugar. Rate Your Plate is a method that helps you judge your food portions. In fact, Rate Your Plate gives you portion power. For most people with type 2 diabetes, eating smaller portions makes their blood sugar go down. Here's how Rate Your Plate works. After you've put your food on your plate, take a look.

- Is about one-fourth of your plate filled with starchy foods, such as noodles, rice, corn, peas, or potatoes?
- Is about one-fourth of your plate filled with main dish (protein) foods, such as meat, poultry, fish, or meat substitutes, such as cheese, eggs, or tofu?
- Is at least half of your plate filled with vegetables, such as salad, or cooked vegetables like carrots, green beans, spinach, or sliced tomatoes?
- You may also want to add one or two side foods along with your meal, such as a dinner roll and a small piece of fruit.

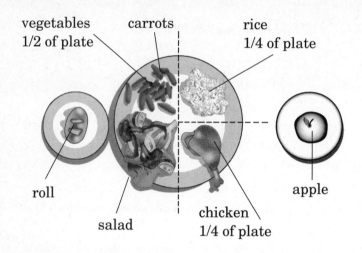

vegetables
1/2 of plate

carrots

rice
1/4 of plate

roll

apple

salad

chicken
1/4 of plate

Check your plate against the picture shown above. How did you do? What changes do you think you need to make?

- Do you need to work on including more vegetables or fruit?
- Do you need to cut back on starches?
- I'll work on_____this week.

Now you know how to Rate Your Plate. Other members of your family who don't have diabetes but want to lose weight might want to rate their plates along with you. Your family is a key part of your diabetes team when it comes to food and meal planning. Lean on them. Ask them for help and support. You may also become a role model for your family and friends by rating your plate and using portion power. Rate Your Plate works great when you're eating out. For more on eating out, see Chapter 5.

Now let's talk about another diabetes meal planning method you can use before you see a dietitian. It's called Carbohydrate Counting.

Carbohydrate Counting

We've talked about portion power when you Rate Your Plate. Now we're going to talk about portion power with a focus on carbohydrates.

Carbohydrate counting is also called by a shorter name, Carb Counting. By counting carbohydrates, or carbs, in the foods you eat, you'll have another way to keep your blood sugar on track. All foods contain the nutrients that your body needs: carbohydrate, protein, and fat.

- **Carbohydrate.** Carbohydrate foods can be put into four groups:

  1. Starches, such as crackers, cereal, corn, bread, rice, and tortillas
  2. Fruits, such as berries, cherries, mangos, and peaches
  3. Milk products, such as a cup of milk, yogurt, or buttermilk
  4. Sweets and desserts, such as cookies, cake, ice cream, and pastries

- **Protein.** Protein foods can be put into two groups:

  1. Meats, such as beef, pork, fish, or chicken
  2. Meat substitutes, such as beans, cheese, eggs, or tofu

- **Fat.** Fats include cream cheese, salad dressing, margarine, butter, mayonnaise, and oil.

Carbs give you calories and energy. But they also raise your blood sugar more than anything else you eat. Protein and fat give you calories and energy, too, but they don't raise your blood sugar. (If you need to lose weight, though, using portion power for protein foods and fats will help you.)

Most people I know are like me—they love carb foods. And many carb foods are healthy foods. Carbs provide good taste, pleasure, energy, vitamins, minerals, and fiber. Even though carbs raise blood sugar more than other foods, it's important for you to have some carbohydrates. For many reasons, then, "carbs count." If you can get the right balance between the amount of carbs you eat and your insulin or diabetes pills, that will help keep your blood sugar in your target range.

For many people, having

- 3 or 4 servings of carbs at each meal and
- 1 or 2 carb servings at snacks

is about right. Then round out your meal with:

- 1 serving of meat, fish, or poultry
- plenty of colorful veggies, such as green beans, broccoli, red peppers, or cabbage. For people with type 2 diabetes, you can eat as much as you want of non-starchy vegetables that are raw or made without fat.
- healthy fats, such as canola oil, olive oil, nuts, seeds, or avocado.

Here is a meal that has four carb choices. The carb choices are in **bold** print so you can see them.

- **3 small corn tortillas** (3 carbs) with meat, salsa, lettuce, and chopped tomato
- **1/3 cup of rice** (1 carb)

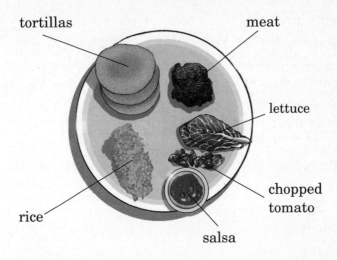

But what about portion sizes for carbs? Portion power with carbs helps keep your blood sugar in your target range. And by keeping your blood sugars in your target range, you can prevent or delay diabetes problems.

Take a look at the serving size guide below.

Carb Choice	Serving Size	Example (each has 15 grams of carbs)
Bread	1 slice	1 small tortilla
Starchy side dishes		
rice or noodles	1/3 cup	1/3 cup spaghetti
corn	1/2 cup	1/2 large ear of corn
Fruit	1/2 cup or 1 piece	1 small apple
Milk	1 cup (8 ounces)	1 small carton
Sweets	2-inch square	1 small piece of cake
	Amount to equal 15 grams of carbs (check the food label)	2 small cookies

Earlier I mentioned that my mom has diabetes. In 2003, after Thanksgiving, she was diagnosed. Mama was having severe back problems and wasn't able to be very active. But she and my dad were still enjoying the holidays with more food, which meant more calories. As a result her weight went up to its highest point ever. As part of a routine checkup, her doctor checked her blood sugar. Her blood sugar level indicated she might have diabetes, so her doctor checked again a week later. Her blood sugar was still too high. Mama was scared when she was diagnosed with diabetes. She was scared because her sister had died from diabetes problems. But she was also surprised. She said she never thought she would have to worry about diabetes—even though diabetes ran in her family.

Her doctor signed her up for diabetes education classes at one of the local hospitals. While she was waiting to attend the classes and see a dietitian, she wanted me to be her dietitian! She wanted to get started right away. I told her it would be hard to be her daughter and her dietitian at the same time. She needed her own dietitian. But while she was waiting to see the dietitian, we got started. She and I talked about Rate Your Plate. After rating her own dinner plate, she decided she was eating way too many carbs. Mama loves carbs like I do—like mother like daughter, they always say. She also knew she and her doctor had agreed that she'd work on losing 15 pounds. We then talked about carb counting and trying for three carb choices at each meal and one carb choice for an evening snack.

Mama wanted her carb counting to be as simple as possible. She didn't want to be looking things up in a book all the time. Here's what we worked out for her to count as one carb choice:

1/2 cup of any starchy food, such as potatoes, cooked beans, peas, or corn

1/3 cup of pasta or rice

1 small piece of fruit or 1/2 cup of fruit

1 cup of milk or yogurt

1/2 cup of low-fat ice cream or frozen yogurt

1 small cookie

1 handful (about 3/4 ounce) of pretzels, baked chips, or snack crackers

1 small dinner roll, tortilla, or muffin

1 piece of bread, 1 biscuit, 1/2 English muffin, 1/2 hamburger or hot dog bun, or 1/4 of a bakery bagel

1 cup of soup, such as chicken noodle, tomato, or split pea

1/2 cup of cooked cereal, such as oatmeal or grits

3/4 cup of dry ready-to-eat cereal, such as Cheerios

Any food that contains about 15 grams of total carbohydrate on the Nutrition Facts Label (see page 14)

Mama thought the serving sizes seemed awfully small, especially that one-fourth of a bagel. Then we talked about having three carb choices at breakfast. Three carbs could be half of a bagel (two carb choices) and a 1/2 cup orange juice (one carb choice) to drink with her medicine. That seemed more like something she could do.

Next we did some meal planning for lunch and dinner. She decided on a sandwich on whole wheat bread (two carb choices), and some baked chips (one carb choice) for lunch. For dinner she wanted all three of her carb choices as spaghetti (about 1 cup).

Nutrition Facts

Serving Size: 3/4 cup (30g; 1.1 oz)
Servings Per Container: About 12

Amount Per Serving

Calories 110   **Calories From Fat** 5

Total Fat 0.5g	
Saturated Fat 0g	
Cholesterol 0mg	
Sodium 20mg	
Potassium 120mg	
Total Carbohydrates 25g	
Dietary Fiber 2g	
Sugars 2g	
Protein 2g	

For her bedtime snack, Mama said she would have a piece of fruit (one carb choice), like a peach, apple, or orange. Or she might choose a glass of 1% milk for one carb. Or she might have a cup of light yogurt, like lemon or blackberry, for one carb. Or a small cookie would be one carb.

"This isn't so hard," Mama said. "It's like I have a bank account of carbs for my meals and my evening snack. Then I spend the carbs in my bank account for the foods I love."

Then she thought about the rest of her meals. "But what about the rest of my meal?" Mama asked. "What about the meat and my salad with dressing?" I suggested she try for about six ounces of lean meat, poultry, or fish each day.

"I don't love meat the way I love carbs, but I'm not sure how much six ounces a day would be," Mama said. "And I need this to be simple. I don't have all day to be weighing and measuring my food. Besides, I thought you said carbs were what would raise my blood sugar."

"That's right, carbohydrates are what raise blood sugar, but because you want to lose weight, you'll want to watch your portions of meats, too," I said.

"So portion power is coming into play with meats, too," Mama said. "How can I keep this simple?" We decided to look at a serving of three ounces of fish, poultry, or meat this way:

- a meat patty or serving the size of a mayonnaise jar lid
- a serving the size of the palm of your hand
- a serving the size of a deck of cards
- three meatballs the size of ping pong balls or golf balls
- a serving the size of a check book.

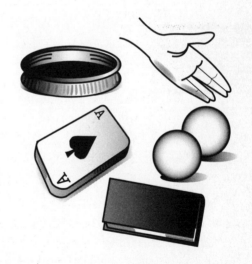

"Those would all fill about one-fourth of my plate, just like when I rate my plate," Mama said. "That makes sense to me. But what about tuna fish or cottage cheese—how do you count them?" she asked. We decided to count half of a 6-ounce can of water-packed tuna or 3/4 cup of low-fat cottage cheese the same as 3 ounces of meat.

"But what about regular cheese—how do I count it?" Mama asked.

"Mama," I said, "one slice of cheese would be equal to 1 ounce of protein. Or a 1-inch cube of cheese, say the size of four dice, would be equal to 1 ounce of meat. You know that a lot of cheeses are high in fat and cholesterol. Think about choosing fat-free or low-fat cheeses when you can. This will be good for your cholesterol level."

"That reminds me that we haven't talked about fats yet, like margarine and oils," Mama said. "I know they say to eat less fat to lose weight."

"That's right, Mama," I said. "Fats have twice as many calories as carbs or protein. So choosing one or two fats at a meal or snack would be about the right amount."

"So how much is a fat?" Mama asked. "And keep it simple."

"A fat serving is about five grams of fat and about 45 calories, but that's not simple, is it?" I said. Mama and I decided about four fats a day would be right for her, and that she'd count as a fat:

- 1 teaspoon margarine, butter, mayonnaise, or oil. That's about the size of the tip of your thumb.
- 1 tablespoon reduced-fat margarine, reduced-fat mayonnaise, salad dressing, cream cheese, or half-and-half cream, the size of the pad of your thumb.
- 2 tablespoons reduced-fat salad dressing, reduced-fat cream cheese, or reduced-fat sour

cream. Two tablespoons would be about half a ladle of dressing at a salad bar.

"How would you like some good news, Mama?" I asked.

"What's good about having diabetes?" she asked.

"The good news is that sometimes finding out you have diabetes is a wake-up call," I said. "People eat better, lose weight, get more active, start feeling better, and just enjoy life more. But the best news about diabetes is that you can prevent or delay diabetes problems like the problems Aunt Carla had."

"That is the best news I've had in a long time!" Mama said. "Is that all there is to eating with diabetes?"

"That's a good start, Mama," I said. "Plus just keep on making healthy food choices."

The time had arrived for Mama's diabetes education classes. I told Mama that she needed to tell her dietitian the way she likes to eat and then work together to design her own meal plan.

Your meal plan needs to fit your schedule, your likes and dislikes in foods, how active you are, when you like to eat, and where you go when you eat out. You and your dietitian will then design a meal plan that will fit the way you live and will include the foods you and your family like.

Luckily, a diabetes meal plan is good for the whole family. Making one dinner is hard, but making two—one for you and one for your family— just won't work. The foods you choose for taking care of your diabetes are the same foods that we all need to eat to stay healthy, whether we have diabetes or not. It's been great that Dad has been part of Mama's diabetes team. He's helping her count carbs. In fact, he's lost about 10 pounds by rating his plate and counting his carbs, too. And he's starting to walk some. Mama has been a good role model for him.

The first day of Mama's classes, a nurse educator talked to the group about diabetes in general, about checking blood sugar, and about things that affect blood sugar. Many family members, like me, were there to learn about diabetes care. They asked lots of questions and learned from each other.

Mama then worked with Marion, a dietitian and CDE. Marion started by talking about Carb Counting with Mama. Marion was pleased to learn that Mama had already started counting her carbs. Marion agreed that three carb choices at meals and one carb choice for a bedtime snack was a good starting point for Mama. Marion told Mama the next step was to start checking her blood sugar to see how this plan was working for her. For more on checking your blood sugar, see Chapter 7.

Marion gave Mama more information about using the food label for Carb Counting:

Steps in Using a Food Label

1. Look first at the serving size. All of the numbers in the Nutrition Facts box are based on this serving size. Is this the serving size you will be eating? How many servings are in the container or bag?
2. Look at the total carbohydrate. How many grams of carbohydrate are there in one serving?

Nutrition Facts

Serving Size 1 cup (58g)
Servings Per Container about 8

Amount Per Serving	Multi-Bran Chex	with 1/2 cup skim milk
Calories	200	240
Calories from Fat	15	15
	% Daily Value**	
Total Fat 1.5g*	**2%**	**3%**
Saturated Fat 0g	**0%**	**0%**
Polyunsaturated Fat 0.5g		
Monounsaturated Fat 0g		
Cholesterol 0mg	**0%**	**1%**
Sodium 380mg	**16%**	**19%**
Potassium 220mg	**6%**	**12%**
Total Carbohydrate 49g	**16%**	**18%**
Dietary Fiber 8g	**30%**	**30%**
Sugars 12g		
Other Carbohydrate 29g		
Protein 4g		

3. Divide total grams of carbohydrate by 15 to find out the number of carb servings. Or you can use this chart to find out the number of carb choices or servings:

Total Carbohydrates in Grams	Count as
0–5	Do not count
6–10	1/2 carb serving
11–20	1 carb serving
21–25	1 1/2 carb servings
26–35	2 carb servings

Marion, the dietitian, and Mama then talked about making healthy food choices when planning meals. Marion suggested eating a wide variety of foods every day. Marion said this meant:

- Eating some fruit each day.

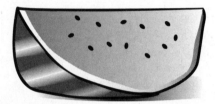

- Eating lots of vegetables that aren't starchy, such as tomatoes, green beans, cabbage, asparagus, cauliflower, green beans, broccoli, carrots, mushrooms, okra, leafy greens, and turnips.

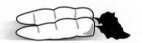

- Trying to eat different colored fruits and vegetables, such as dark green (collards or broccoli), orange (cantaloupe, apricots, or carrots), red (watermelon or tomatoes), blue (blueberries), and white (banana, cauliflower, or turnips). Some people call this "eating the rainbow." Research shows that eating colorful fruits and veggies also helps prevent cancer and heart disease.

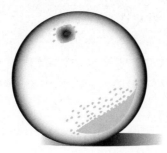

- Choosing different kinds of starches, such as corn tortillas, black or pinto beans, hominy, whole-grain breakfast cereals and breads, and sweet potatoes.
- Eating high-fiber foods, like beans, whole-grain breads and cereals, and fruits and vegetables.
- Checking food labels for breakfast cereals that have at least four grams of fiber per serving.
- Looking for breads that have two to three grams of fiber per slice.
- Choosing dairy products that are low in fat. Fat-free milk and 1% milk are the good choices. Light yogurts are also great when you want something sweet.

Mama and Marion decided to choose only one or two changes for Mama to work on. Mama decided she wanted to eat more colorful fruits and vegetables. She thought it sounded like fun to eat the rainbow.

You may want to think about doing some of these things—one at a time—along with rating your plate or carb counting. Read through the list of ideas above and pick one action item you want to work on.

I'll work on _____
this week.

I'll work on _____
the following week.

Marion gave Mama a longer list of carb choices. That list is at the end of this book in the section called Diabetes Tools. If you decide to count your carbs, this longer list may come in handy later on.

Glycemic Index

Mama heard about the glycemic index on TV. The glycemic index is a number that tells how much a carb food will raise blood sugar for some people: a lot, a little, or somewhere in between.

Mama called and said, "I'm confused by this glycemic index. I thought all carbs raised blood sugar."

"You're right," I said. "All carbs do raise blood sugar, but some carbs raise blood sugar levels more than others. For example, corn flakes raise blood sugar more than oatmeal. For some people using the glycemic index can help keep their blood sugar on target."

"Well, what carbs raise blood sugar less?" Mama asked.

"The glycemic index for a food is not the same for everyone. The glycemic index of a food is also not the same for every meal. It depends on what else is in the meal. It also depends on how well a food is cooked, like how long you cook your pasta. But you may have lower blood sugars after eating a meal if you choose

- dense and chewy breads rather than white bread.
- breakfast cereals made with oats, barley, or bran. Oatmeal or all-bran cereals raise blood sugar less than cornflakes or toasted rice cereals.
- pasta more often than potatoes. Cooking pasta for shorter times, sometimes called al dente, keeps blood sugars down more than soft overcooked pasta.
- converted rice or long grain rice. They raise blood sugar a little less than short grain rice.
- milk and yogurt.
- plenty of non-starchy veggies and fruits.
- pinto, navy, lima, or kidney beans as well as chickpeas and lentils.
- sweet potatoes. They raise blood sugar less than white potatoes.
- new potatoes. They raise blood sugar less than baked or mashed potatoes.

"It's best to choose the carbs you love so you feel satisfied. When you can, eat the carb foods that raise blood sugar less. Since you like oatmeal, Mama, having it a few times a week may help your blood sugar level. Since you like them, include pinto and navy beans instead of potatoes when it works into your meal.

"The glycemic index is just another tool that you can use to keep your blood sugar in your target range after meals."

Rate Your Plate or Carb Counting works for most of my clients. Take Michael, for instance. He was 18 years old when I first started working with him. His doctor referred Michael to me because his blood fats and blood sugar were both too high. Michael didn't have diabetes, but he did have pre-diabetes. Pre-diabetes is the condition that comes before diabetes. It means that blood sugar levels are higher than normal but aren't high enough to be called diabetes. Like many people, Michael had pre-diabetes and didn't know it until he saw his doctor and had his blood sugar checked. People with pre-diabetes might get type 2 diabetes soon or later on.

Michael had a number of risks for diabetes:

- Diabetes ran in his family.
- He was very inactive.
- He had gained weight.

Michael had played football and even worked out at the school gym. Then he had an injury and couldn't play football anymore. He stopped going to the gym, and his weight went up. When he went to the doctor for his college physical, he found out he had pre-diabetes and high blood fats. Michael was shocked. He knew his grandparents had diabetes. And he knew about the problems that diabetes can bring on. His grandmother had eye and kidney problems from her diabetes. And his grandfather had foot problems from his type 2 diabetes. But Michael was surprised about having pre-diabetes, because he was so young. After all, he was only 18 years old and just getting ready to go to college.

For Michael's visit with me, I asked him to bring a record of everything he ate and drank for three days. Here's how it went:

Michael also said, "I tend to eat a good amount when I go out to eat. There's usually nothing left on my plate. I'm also crazy with sauces, catsup, and gravies. I put them on everything.

"I also like to eat fast food, like the meatball sub I had at lunch yesterday," Michael said. "I will sometimes super size my meal to get a bigger serving of fries and a larger drink."

Michael's Food Record

Breakfast—Large bowl of cereal with whole milk, 2–3 cups apple juice

Lunch—Large meatball sub, chips, large soda

Snack—Frozen waffle with peanut butter and lots of syrup, big glass of milk

Dinner—Barbequed ribs, potato salad, baked beans

Snack—Bag of microwave popcorn with a large soda

Michael wanted to make changes to prevent getting type 2 diabetes and to lose weight for college. We talked about Rating Your Plate and Carb Counting. He decided he wanted to rate his plate. He also wanted to start going to the gym again.

He still wanted to eat out with his friends. We talked about picking lower-calorie choices when he was eating out. Michael decided he'd choose smaller portions and not super size his meals. He decided to drink diet soft drinks.

Michael and I reviewed the difference in calories and fat when he switched from a meatball sub to a turkey sub:

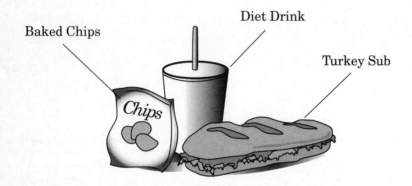

"Wow!" Michael said. "I never dreamed I could save 600 calories by switching from the meatball sub to the turkey sub and by choosing baked chips and a diet drink. That's a painless change I can make right away."

Michael did well. In three months, he had lost 10 pounds and was at the goal weight he had set for himself. And his blood sugar and cholesterol were back in the normal range.

Michael said, "I'm going to keep watching what I eat and being active. I really enjoy feeling and looking better. And I want to beat the odds and keep from getting type 2 diabetes."

Chapter 4

Meal Planning and Shopping

We plan so many things in our lives. We make to-do lists to get things done. We make plans to see our friends on Friday night. We visit with our family on Sundays. We plan birthday parties for friends and family. We plan fishing trips.

But many people I work with never plan meals. They spend a lot of time stopping at the grocery store to pick up something for dinner. Or they might pick up carry-out or fast food.

Planning your meals is a helpful tool whether you have diabetes or not. Meal planning helps in many ways:

- We can plan meals that will include the foods we love.
- We can plan meals that follow our meal plan.
- We can plan meals that contain low-fat protein sources, such as lean chops, chicken breasts, fish, shellfish, and roasts.
- We can plan meals that include fruits and vegetables, with all the colors of the rainbow.
- We can plan meals that will save money and time!

So how does meal planning work? Here are the steps that many of my clients use for successful meal planning:

- Use a calendar or a form for each week. There's a form that you can use in the Diabetes Tools section at the back of this book. A sample of a completed form appears at the end of this chapter.
- First fill in your schedule for the week. You may have a support group on Wednesday nights. Write that in. If you're having lunch with a friend on Monday, write that down. If you have a diabetes visit with your health care team on Thursday at 2:00 P.M., write that in. If you're having a friend over for a meal, write that in. And so on. In other words, write in all of your plans for the week.
- Next, plan your meals and snacks for each day, taking into account your schedule for the week. You may have quick breakfasts during the week, like ready-to-eat cereal with fresh fruit or an English muffin with a tablespoon of peanut butter and a banana. On Saturday, you may plan a breakfast that takes more time, like eggs and toast. On Sunday you might eat a bagel with low-fat cream cheese.
- Next, plan your lunches. Perhaps you want to use foods you can carry with you for lunch, like a turkey sandwich on whole-wheat pita bread, baked chips, raw veggies, and an apple. Or you may want to plan a main course salad for lunch one day. It might be a taco salad using leftover chicken and beans with salad greens and other veggies. Top it with salsa or salsa mixed with

low-fat French dressing. If you plan to purchase lunch, write that on your calendar.

- It's a good idea to plan foods for your snacks so you'll have foods you enjoy and that match your meal plan. Your snack could be low-fat or fat-free cheese with a pear, pretzels, graham crackers, or a light yogurt.
- Now to dinners. If you have a support group meeting at night, you may want to purchase a main course frozen dinner that can be prepared quickly. Add a vegetable and a whole-grain roll for a complete meal. Write that onto your calendar. Other nights you may want to make a simple and fast meal of a baked potato topped with low-fat canned chili or a baked potato topped with cottage cheese and salsa. All you need to go with these meals is frozen broccoli or some other frozen vegetable you like or maybe a salad. Think about the bags of pre-washed salad greens to save time.
- Plan for leftovers. When you grill chicken and vegetables, make extras for lunch or another night later on. If you have a casserole, make two and freeze one. It will taste great in a month.
- Think about trying a new recipe every week or so. This keeps your meals interesting. This can also keep you from feeling deprived or bored with your meals.
- After you have your weekly menu planned, it's time to make your shopping list. Take into account what you already have on hand. Check your cupboards and freezer to see what you might want to use this week. Maybe use up the pork roast or the chicken breasts that are in the

freezer? What about the pasta in the cupboard or the canned tuna? Now make your shopping list. There's a shopping list form in the Diabetes Tools section at the end of this book. It may be helpful. Or just make your own list on a piece of paper. Write down the items you need to buy for the week. You might need fresh or frozen vegetables, fruit, milk, yogurt, bread, frozen dinners, chicken breasts, deli meats, low-fat cheese, and snack foods.

- If you like, you can use the bottom of the Meal Planning form in the Diabetes Tools section to keep track of your activities for the week. Writing down your biking or whatever you like to do makes you feel good about yourself. It also helps to keep you moving!

- As you run out of food items over the week, keep a running list of items you need to pick up. This list might include mustard, canned soups, chicken broth, canned tomatoes, or tuna fish.

- When you do your shopping, you'll know exactly what you need to buy for the week. You'll be able go through the store more quickly.

- To save money, check weekly store sales and coupons. If you need turkey for your lunches but ham is on sale, switch to the ham. If you have a coupon for yogurt, and yogurt is on your list, use the coupon. However, coupons for unhealthy foods or items you may not use aren't a good buy.

- If you rely on your list, you'll save money in another way. You'll only buy what you will use. No more rotting fruits and vegetables that you have to throw away!

Taking time to make a menu and a shopping list will save you time in the long run. You'll already know what you're eating when you get home late and need to make a quick dinner. Not only will your menus match your diabetes meal plan, they will also match your schedule for the week.

My Meal Plans
Week of <u>May 7 to May 13</u>

	Sunday	Monday	Tuesday
Breakfast	1/2 whole-grain bagel 1% milk 1 small apple	Raisin bran 1% milk 1 small apple	Oatmeal 1% milk 1 slice toast
Snack	Small apple	Pretzels	6 ounce container light yogurt
Lunch	Baked chicken Mashed potatoes Green beans	Noon—lunch at Jane's house	Ham sandwich Leftover slaw Baked chips
Snack	3 cups popcorn	15 grapes	1/2 cup light fruit cocktail
Dinner	Chicken sandwich Carrot sticks Baked chips	1 cup chili with beans 1 square cornbread Slaw	Leftover baked chicken 1 cup canned corn Frozen spinach
Snack	1/2 cup pudding	1/2 cup light ice cream	1/2 cup pineapple
	Activity Today	**Activity Today**	**Activity Today**
	Walked 30 minutes at the zoo	Got off bus and walked 5 extra blocks	Walked to post office, 30 minutes

My Meal Plans *continued*

Wednesday	Thursday	Friday	Saturday

English muffin
Peanut butter
Small banana
	Leftover oatmeal
	1 slice whole-
	   wheat toast
	2 tablespoons
	   raisins
		English muffin
		1 slice cheese
		1/2 cup
		   applesauce
			Scrambled eggs
			1 slice whole-
			   wheat toast
			1/2 grapefruit

3 graham crackers	Orange	2 bread sticks	1/2 cup Cheerios

1 can chicken
   noodle soup
Crackers
Pear
	1 cup leftover
	   chili with beans
	Crackers
	Carrot sticks
		Frozen dinner
		Whole-wheat roll
			2 slices cheese
			Toast
			Baked chips
			Celery sticks

6 ounce
   container light
   yogurt
	2 pm—see
	   Dr. Wood
	Apple
		6 crackers	Fudgesicle

7:30 pm—
   support group
Frozen dinner
Frozen mixed
   veggies
Dinner roll
	Whole-wheat
	   pita bread
	Baked chips
	Sliced tomatoes
		7 pm—Robert
		   over for dinner
		Pork chops
		Baked potato
		Salad
		Fresh mixed fruit
			Grilled sirloin
			Rice
			Salad
			Green beans
			Watermelon

Orange	2 small cookies	1/2 cup light
		   yogurt
			3 cups popcorn
			   at the movie

Activity Today	**Activity Today**	**Activity Today**	**Activity Today**

None	Worked out at
	   the gym after
	   seeing
	   Dr. Wood,
	   1 hour
		Ran errands
		   and walked
		   at lunch,
		   30 minutes
			Walked
			   30 minutes
			   while shopping
			   at the mall

Chapter 5

Tips for Eating Out with Diabetes

I'm old enough to remember when eating out was something special. It was someone's birthday or it was when Aunt Betty came to visit.

Eating away from home isn't anything special anymore. A few of my clients eat out for all their meals. Others eat out six to ten times a week. What's the problem with eating out? Here's my short list:

- Even though we eat out a lot, many of us still think it's a special treat and eat more than usual.
- To make things taste great and keep us coming back, chefs use more fat and sauces than we do at home. More fat means more calories.
- Portions of foods served in restaurants are getting bigger and bigger.
- Fast food places try to make us think it's a better deal to "super size" our meal and then we overeat.
- Fruits and vegetables are hard to find when we eat out.
- Desserts are sometimes big enough to serve four people!

Everyone loves to eat out. It's a way of life. It's how we get to see our friends and family. How often do we say, "Let's get together for lunch!"?

So let's tackle eating out step-by-step.

Top Tips for Eating Away from Home

1. Try to eat out no more than three times a week. You'll save calories and money.
2. Know your meal plan or write it down. How many carbs do you plan to eat?
3. Plan ahead. Think about what you'll order and how much you'll eat.
4. Call if you're unsure of the menu. If you're not sure that you'll find the type of foods you want to order, go someplace else.
5. Work with your server. Here are some things you may want to ask:

   - How is the fish cooked? Is it grilled or fried?
   - Is there a sauce? Think about all the times you've been surprised by a sauce not mentioned on the menu.
   - Can you get a baked potato instead of fries?
   - Can you get the baked potato toppings, such as butter or sour cream, on the side?
   - Can you get salad dressings on the side?
   - If you made it clear you wanted your salad dressing or the sauce on the side and your plate arrives with your food swimming in sauce, send it back!

6. When your food arrives, compare it to your goals for the meal. How many carbs are in the rice? If

there are two chicken breasts or two chops,
think about taking one of them home for
tomorrow's lunch, along with the extra rice.

7. Add sauces and salad dressings one of two ways:

   - Dip the tines of your fork into the sauce or
     dressing. Then spear a piece of meat or lettuce
     for a little sauce or dressing with each bite.
   - Add 1 teaspoon of dressing or sauce at a time.
     When you've eaten that, add another tea-
     spoon.

   You'll eat less salad dressing or sauce using
   either of these methods.

8. At a fast food place, ask them to leave off the
   mayo or sauces on sandwiches and ask for a
   packet of mustard, catsup, or barbeque sauce.
   You'll eat fewer calories and fat.

9. Stick with grilled, broiled, or baked fish, poultry,
   and meat.

10. Remove the skin from poultry. Trim fat off
    meats.

11. Order the smallest size of meat, such as a
    4-ounce filet rather than a 12-ounce piece of
    prime rib. Besides having portion power, the
    filet will be lower in fat and calories.

12. Split an entree with a family member or friend.
    You'll eat less and save money, too.

13. Order two appetizers instead of a main course.

14. Don't forget about the bread basket or the
    tortilla basket. Can you eat just one piece of
    bread and count it as one of your carb choices?
    Or about 15 tortilla chips? Will this carb choice
    fit into the rest of the meal you've ordered?

If not, move the basket away from you or ask your server to take it away.

15. Use small amounts of fats like oil and butter. Or don't add extra. The chef has already added more than you or I can even guess.
16. If you want to Rate Your Plate, check the size of the plate when you eat out. Sometimes the plates are more like platters. Check the amount of food and ask for a box to take any extra food home for a later meal. Studies show that the more we're served, the more we eat.
17. Split sweets and treats with a friend or family member. Order one dessert and four spoons!

This is a long list of tips for eating away from home. Pick one tip to work on. When you have mastered it, pick one or two more to try.

When I eat out this week, I'll _____.

When I eat out next week, I'll _____.

Chapter 6

What to Eat When You're Sick

Like everyone else, people with diabetes get sick. They get colds, the flu, or an upset stomach. When you get sick, take extra care of yourself to keep your blood sugar levels in your target range.

Work with your health care team to design your sick day plan. Until you do, here are some tips you can use for sick days:

Tips for Sick Days

- Check your blood sugar every four hours and write down the results.
- Check your temperature when you check your blood sugar.
- Drink plenty of fluids. If your temperature is over 99 degrees, drink some fluids every hour.
- Take your diabetes medicines. An illness can make your blood sugar go up.

  - Take your usual diabetes pills, except for the pills you take only when you eat.
  - If you use insulin, take your usual dose.

- Eat your usual amount of carbohydrates in your meal plan.

  - If you have an upset stomach or are vomiting, try to take enough fluids that contain carbs to equal the carbohydrates in your meal plan. Space the fluids out over the day. Taking a few sips every 15 minutes may help keep fluids down. Often sodas, such as ginger ale, help with nausea, and they contain carbohydrates.
  - If you have a sore throat, try soft foods, such as yogurt, to get your carbohydrates in a way that won't hurt your throat.

Liquid and Soft Sick Day Foods

The foods listed below each have about 15 grams of carbohydrate and can be used in your meal plan when you are sick with a cold, flu, or upset stomach or when you have dental work. The amount of food can be doubled or tripled if you need more carbohydrates for your meal plan.

15 gram Carb Foods	Amount
Regular (not diet) soft drink	1/2 cup
Juices	1/2 cup
Sports drink	1 cup
Milk	1 cup
Yogurt, plain or light	1 cup
Chocolate milk	1/2 cup
Milk shake	1/2 cup

(continued)

15 gram Carb Foods	Amount
Regular (not diet) Jell-O	1/2 cup
Fruit cup	1/2 cup
Applesauce	1/2 cup
Banana	1 small
Cooked cereal	1/2 cup
Mashed potatoes	1/2 cup
Rice	1/3 cup
Cream or tomato soup (made with water)	1 cup
Cream or tomato soup (made with milk)	1/2 cup
Chicken noodle or chicken rice soup	1 cup
Crackers	6–8
Toast	1 slice
Pudding, regular	1/4 cup
Pudding, sugar-free	1/2 cup
Ice cream	1/2 cup
Frozen yogurt	1/2 cup
Sherbet or sorbet	1/4 cup
Fruit juice bars, frozen	1 bar
Jam or jelly	1 tablespoon
Honey	1 tablespoon
Sugar	1 tablespoon

Talk with your health care team about when to call if you're sick. Write down the phone numbers that you would call during the day and at night.

Daytime telephone number:_____

Evening telephone number: _____

In the meantime, here are some general ideas of when to call.

When to Call Your Health Care Team

Call right away if you're

- having blood sugar levels over 300.
- vomiting or have diarrhea for more than a day.
- running a high fever for more than a day. A high fever is over 101 degrees.
- sick for more than two days.
- unable to eat for more than one day.

When you call your health care provider, be ready to give these facts:

- How long you've been sick: _____

- Your blood sugar levels: _____

- Your temperature: _____

- Medicines you're taking: _____

- How much you've been able to eat and drink:

  _____

- Your symptoms: _____

- Your pharmacist's phone number: _____

  It's a good idea to know of a pharmacy that is open all night and on weekends: _____

After talking with your health care team about your own plan for when you're sick, write below the reasons your health care team says you need to call.

Reasons to call my diabetes health care team:

- _____
- _____
- _____
- _____
- _____
- _____
- _____
- _____

Feeling Bad: A Real Life Story

Robert had a bad cough, sore throat, and runny nose that kept getting worse. His blood sugar levels were getting higher and higher, too. He went to the drugstore and bought some cough syrup and some cold pills. After two days of not getting better and running a fever, he called his health care team.

Robert reported

- three days of being sick.
- blood sugars of 200 in the mornings, and in the 300s during the day.
- a temperature of 100.
- taking his diabetes, blood pressure, and cholesterol medicines plus cough syrup and cold pills.
- eating soft foods and liquids to get all the carbs in his meal plan.

- a very sore throat, bad cough, runny nose, and not sleeping.

Robert was given an appointment for that afternoon. Robert took his logbook of his blood sugar readings and the medicines he had been taking with him. His team checked his blood pressure, temperature, and blood sugar and listened to his heart and his breathing. Robert had bronchitis (brong-KI-tis) and needed an antibiotic. The doctor raised his insulin dose to get his blood sugar levels down. He also told Robert to keep eating all the carbs in his meal plan and to drink plenty of fluids. His team said to call if he didn't feel better in a day or so. He was also to call if his blood sugars didn't drop after the added insulin.

After 10 days, Robert was his old self. The cough was gone, his breathing was normal, and he was hungry and ate his full meal plan. Robert's team asked him to continue to check his blood sugar levels more often for another few days after he went back to his regular dose of insulin.

Chapter 7

Checking Your Blood Sugar

Keeping your blood sugar close to your target range is your best route for good health. You'll feel better, too. Checking your blood sugar is the only way to know how your blood sugar is doing.

Some people with diabetes think they can guess when their blood sugar is high or low. But studies show they're wrong most of the time when they just guess.

You can keep track of your blood sugar level in two ways:

1. Use a meter to check your blood sugar. This gives you a snapshot of your blood sugar level at that moment. Your diabetes team will teach you how to check.
2. Ask your doctor or nurse to order an A-1-C (A-one-see) check several times a year. An A-1-C check is a special blood sugar test "with a memory." The A-1-C check tells you your average blood sugar for the past two to three months.

By using your results from both of these checks, you and your diabetes team will know how your diabetes plan is working. These checks will also help you and your diabetes team know when to make changes in your diabetes plan.

At Mama's second diabetes education class, a nurse gave her a meter and showed her how to check her blood sugar. The nurse explained to Mama that blood sugar levels go up and down all day long. The nurse said, "Checking blood sugar any time and any place and keeping track of the results will help you know what's going on with your blood sugar. You'll see what food, exercise, stress, and medicine do to your blood sugar levels."

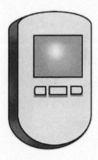

Sometimes it's tricky to learn how to use a meter. When Mama got home from her class, she tried to check her blood sugar. Her meter kept giving her an error message, so she knew something wasn't right. She called me, but I wasn't at home. She called the diabetes educator, but she had left for the day. She then called her pharmacist who had sold her the strips she needed for her meter. The pharmacist went through the steps for her meter with Mama. Always remember that you have many members on your diabetes team—your doctor, dietitian, nurse, and pharmacist and your family and friends. Don't be afraid to ask them to help when you have a problem. Also, most meter companies have toll-free customer service numbers you can call for help. Some meters come with a video that shows how to use your meter.

Mama now checks her blood sugar without any problems. She likes seeing how the foods she eats affect her blood sugar. She also likes seeing how much walking or yard work lowers her blood sugar level.

It's a good idea to have your nurse or dietitian watch as you check your blood sugar using your meter. Then you'll know your meter is giving you the right blood sugar readings.

How Often Do I Check My Blood Sugar?

Many people check their blood sugar several times a day—before or after meals and before bedtime. Talk with your diabetes team about when and how often to check your blood sugar. Then write down the times to check in your logbook or here, as a reminder:

I need to check my blood sugar at least _____ times a
    day.
I need to check my blood sugar:

  ☐ when I get up in the morning
  ☐ two hours after meals
  ☐ two hours after snacks

In the beginning, Mama's doctor wanted her to check her blood sugar twice a day and at different times of the day. He also asked Mama to write down her blood sugar results in a logbook he gave her.

BLOOD SUGAR RECORD

	BREAKFAST		LUNCH		DINNER		BEDTIME	
	before	after	before	after	before	after	before	after
MON.								
TUE.								
WED.								
THU.								
FRI.								
SAT.								
SUN.								

If you need a logbook, look in the Diabetes Tools section at the end of this book. There's a log sheet you can copy into a notebook or you can copy it on a copy machine.

One morning, Mama checked her blood sugar before she had anything to eat or drink. This is called fasting blood sugar, since she hadn't eaten or drunk anything the night before. That same day Mama checked her blood sugar two hours after she started to eat breakfast. The next day she checked her blood sugar two different times: two hours after she started to eat lunch and two hours after she started to eat her bedtime snack. The next day she checked her blood sugar 1) first thing in the morning and 2) two hours after she started to eat dinner.

At her next doctor visit, Dr. Wood reviewed Mama's blood sugar logbook with her. He said her diabetes plan seemed to be working because her blood sugar levels were within her target range most of the time. Mama's doctor then said she only needed to check her blood sugar a few times a week. But Mama thinks that checking her blood sugar more often and getting feedback help her keep her blood sugar on track.

The A-1-C Check

To be sure her diabetes plan was on target, Mama's doctor also checked her A-1-C, the blood check with a memory, to find out how her average blood sugar had been for the last two to three months. The doctor told Mama that the A-1-C result usually meant this:

If your A-1-C is	Then your average blood sugar was about
6 ⟶	135
7 ⟶	170
8 ⟶	205
9 ⟶	240
10 ⟶	275
11 ⟶	310
12 ⟶	345

"Mrs. Mathews, you're doing a great job," said Dr. Wood. "And your diabetes plan is working well. Your A-1-C is down almost a point. That's very good. Your hard work is paying off. The lower your A-1-C is, the lower your chances are of having any diabetes problems. Let's continue to work toward your A-1-C target of 6."

Look at the chart on the previous page and find your last A-1-C result in the left column and then look across to learn your average blood sugar for the past two to three months. If you don't know your A-1-C, talk with your doctor or nurse to find out your A-1-C result.

The A-1-C checks include all the highs and lows and tell you what your blood sugar levels have been over the last two to three months. You can't get this information from your checks with your blood sugar meter. Your A-1-C result gives you the big picture on how your treatment plan is working. And it's worth repeating that the lower your A-1-C is, the lower your chances are of getting any long-term diabetes problems.

The American Diabetes Association recommends getting your A-1-C checked at least every six months. The higher your A-1-C number, the higher your risk for diabetes problems. If your number is 7 or higher, you may need a change in your diabetes plan to get it lower. Talk with your doctor or health care team.

Dr. Wood said the A-1-C goal for my mom is 6. Talk with your doctor about your A-1-C goal and write it here:

My target for the A-1-C check is _____.

My last A-1-C result was _____.

The American Diabetes Association A-1-C goal is below 7.

Chapter 8

Keeping Your Blood Sugar in Your Target Range

Do you know your blood sugar goals? If you don't, ask your diabetes health care team what yours are. Keeping blood sugar in your target range helps prevent diabetes problems later on, and you'll feel better every day, too. Dr. Wood is following the American Diabetes Association guidelines for his patients. These guidelines are listed below. Your doctor and diabetes team may decide on a different target range for you.

Talk with your diabetes team and set your target blood sugar range, and then fill in the blanks below:

- My blood sugar target before meals and when I wake up:

  _____ to _____
  (American Diabetes Association standard is an average of 90 to 130)

- My blood sugar target two hours after starting to eat a meal:

  Below _____
  (American Diabetes Association standard is below 180)

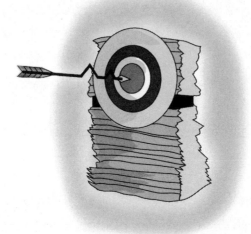

Checking your blood sugar at different times on different days gives you and your diabetes team the big picture of how your diabetes care plan is working. Write down the results and use them to see how food, activity, and stress affect your blood sugar and to look for patterns. Patterns are similar blood sugar results over and over again. If your blood sugar is always high after breakfast or after dinner, talk with your diabetes team about making changes to bring it down.

Chapter 9

What Makes Your Blood Sugar Go Up or Down?

Blood sugar levels rise and fall all day long, every day, for everyone. Your daily checks with your blood sugar meter give you a snapshot of your blood sugar at that moment.

Sometimes your blood sugar checks will show numbers out of your target range. When this happens to my mom, she says, "I don't like it!" Sometimes you know why your blood sugar is lower or higher than your target. Other times, you won't be able to figure it out. Think of blood sugar numbers as clues to what's going on. Take a close look at your blood sugar logbook to see if your blood sugar levels are too high or too low several days in a row at about the same time. This is called a pattern. If the same thing keeps happening over and over again, it might be time to change your diabetes plan. Talk with your diabetes team when you see this happening.

A key to taking care of your diabetes is learning why your blood sugar levels go up and down. If you know the reasons, you can take steps to keep your blood sugar in your target range.

Nathan, one of my clients, used to get high blood sugar after dinner. He said he would get home from work, tired and hungry, and nibble while he was making his dinner. Then he would eat his dinner. When he checked his blood sugar two hours after starting to eat dinner, his blood sugar would be 250 to 300.

Nathan decided he would make extra dinners on the weekend and freeze them. He also bought a supply of frozen dinners to have on hand. "All I have to do is heat something up when I get home," said Nathan. "I also keep fresh veggies handy in case I need a snack before dinner since they don't raise my blood sugar."

Mama found out her blood sugar was higher when she skipped her walks. She also found out it went down when she did extra yard work, like raking leaves or pulling weeds. For more on exercise and diabetes, see Chapter 10.

Nathan takes insulin and diabetes pills for his diabetes. His blood sugar goes up if he forgets to take his diabetes pills. It drops too low when Nathan eats his meals late.

Mama found out that there are many things that can make her blood sugar go up. She was having a bad time with pain in her back. She wasn't able to enjoy her walks. Dr. Wood suggested a new medicine for her back. He warned Mama that the medicine would make her blood sugar go up. Wow, was she surprised when it hit almost 300! Luckily, her blood sugar came down over time—and her back was much better. Now she can enjoy her walks again.

Mama's blood sugar went up for a few reasons. What are they?

- If you guessed her blood sugar went up from being less active, you're right.
- If you guessed her blood sugar went up from the side effects of the new medicine, you're right.
- If you guessed her blood sugar went up from the pain and stress on her body, you're right.

Mama learned that high blood sugars can result from more than one thing at the same time.

My cousin Pam has diabetes. Last year Pam called me because her blood sugar was 285. She also said she was sick with the flu. I told her that being sick raises blood sugar. This year Pam got a flu shot. To learn more about flu shots, see Chapter 11.

Stress will also raise blood sugar. Like many people, Pam has stress at her job. Pam is trying to learn to let go of some things at work that are stressful for her. To learn more about stress and diabetes, see Chapter 15.

So the main things that affect your blood sugar are

- food
- amount of activity
- medicines
- illness
- stress

When your blood sugar is out of your target range, think about the meals and snacks you've eaten or have not eaten. Think about how active you've been. Think about how good or bad you feel. Are you coming down with something? Are you extra stressed or worried about work or something at home? These questions will help solve your blood sugar puzzle.

If Your Blood Sugar Is Too High

If your blood sugar is too high, you may

- be more thirsty than usual
- urinate more often
- have dry or itchy skin
- have more infections
- have cuts or sores that heal more slowly

If your blood sugar is high, ask yourself these questions to figure out the reasons:

- Did I eat my meal or snack on time?
- Did I have a bigger-than-usual meal?
- Did I have a bigger-than-usual snack?
- Did I take my diabetes medicine earlier or later than usual?
- Did I take fewer pills or less insulin than my usual dose?
- Did I forget to take my pills or insulin?
- Did I take other medicines that may have made my blood sugar go up?
- Do I need a higher dose of pills or insulin?
- Do I feel like I'm getting a cold?
- Is my arthritis acting up?
- Was it the minor surgery?
- Was it the dental checkup?

- Am I worried about something?
- How about hormone levels? For more on women's and men's issues related to diabetes, see Chapter 17.

If your blood sugar is too high much of the time, work with your health care team to make changes to your meal plan, activity level, or diabetes medicines. You have the power to make the changes that will work for you.

If Your Blood Sugar Is Too Low

Nathan started to feel shaky and weak. He checked his blood sugar—it was only 60! That's too low. He drank half a cup of juice and that brought his blood sugar level to 75. Nathan didn't know why his blood sugar went low. He asked himself these questions:

- Did I eat enough at my last meal?
- Did I eat earlier than usual?
- Did I skip any meals or snacks today?
- Did I eat enough carbohydrate foods?
- Did I have alcoholic drinks without eating? For more on alcohol and diabetes, see Chapter 18.
- Was I more active than usual today?
- Did I take more diabetes pills or insulin than usual?
- Do I need to reduce the number of pills or amount of insulin I take?

If your blood sugar level goes too low, you can use these same questions to try to find out what happened.

Low blood sugar is also called hypoglycemia (hi-po-gli-see-me-uh), when your blood sugar level drops below 70. People with type 2 diabetes who use meal planning and exercise don't normally get hypoglycemia.

When your blood sugar is this low, you may feel

- anxious
- confused
- dizzy
- grumpy
- hungry
- nervous
- shaky
- sweaty

If you have these feelings and think your blood sugar is too low, use your meter to check your blood sugar level. If you find that your blood sugar is below 70, follow the 15-15 rule. The 15-15 rule reminds you to have 15 grams of carbohydrate and then wait 15 minutes before you check your blood sugar again.

If your blood sugar is still below 70, eat another 15 grams of carbohydrate. You can get about 15 grams of carbohydrate from these things:

- two to five glucose tablets
- 1/2 cup fruit juice
- 1 cup fat-free or 1% milk
- 1/2 cup regular (not diet) soft drink

After 15 minutes, check your blood sugar again. If it's still below 70, have another serving of

15 grams of carbohydrate. Repeat these steps until your blood glucose is above 70.

If your blood sugar is too low too often, you may need a change in your meal plan, your activity, or your diabetes medicines. Keep track of any low blood sugars in your logbook and note the reasons, such as skipping a meal.

Always talk with your diabetes team about blood sugar levels that are too low or too high. Also, talk with your diabetes team about patterns you see in your logbook. You can work with your team to make a change in your diabetes plan.

Now you know that the major factors that can affect your blood sugar are

- food
- exercise
- diabetes medicines
- side effects from other medicines
- being sick
- being stressed
- timing—the times you eat, exercise, and take your diabetes medicines

There are a lot of things that can affect your blood sugar. But checking your blood sugar will help you figure out what's going on. You'll see what food, exercise, stress, and medicines do to your blood sugar levels. You can learn how to use your blood sugar numbers to make changes in your diabetes plan.

Chapter 10

Getting Up and Getting Going

Living an active life is a great way to take care of type 2 diabetes. It's also a great way to delay or prevent type 2 diabetes if you have pre-diabetes.

You don't have to spend hours working out to look and feel better! Just 30 minutes a day will do it. You can even split it into two or three parts. Try a 10-minute walk after every meal. Or think of ways to build extra activity into your day. You don't have to go to a gym unless you want to. Just walk, mop the floor, wash the car, weed the garden, clean the house, or ride your bike. How about dancing? That's fun. Or go swimming. There are many fun things to do to get in motion. The choice is yours.

Exercise helps with type 2 diabetes. Exercise also helps in a lot of other ways:

- It helps relieve stress and promotes calmness.
- It lowers your blood sugar, blood pressure, and blood cholesterol levels.
- It uses up extra sugar in your blood.
- It helps your own insulin work better.
- It makes your heart, muscles, and bones strong.
- It improves your blood flow.

- It tones your muscles.
- It helps you lower your weight and lose inches off your waistline.
- It keeps your body and your joints flexible.
- It burns calories and increases endurance.

So now you know being active helps you lower your blood sugar, blood fats (cholesterol), and blood pressure. It also helps with weight loss. So what are you waiting for? Motion is the potion!

If you haven't been active for a while, check with your health care team first. You may need a checkup before you start being more active.

Here are a few ways to get in motion:

- Walk rather than driving your car or taking the bus.
- Take the stairs.
- Join an exercise group in your area.
- Start a walking group at work or in your neighborhood.
- Do the exercises on TV every morning at home or tape them for later. Exercise videos are ready when you are, too.
- Take a dance class.
- Walk at the mall.
- Walk around while talking on the phone.
- When shopping, take the faraway parking place and walk to the store.
- Carry groceries to your car rather than driving to pick them up.
- Carry things in two trips instead of one.
- Walk to the mailbox or post office.
- Walk the dog after dinner.

- Play with the kids.
- Walk to the drugstore instead of driving or taking the bus.

Pick one thing from the list above to try.

This week, I'll _____.

Next week, I may try_____.

Other things I am thinking of doing are _____

_____.

Mama loves to walk. She walks in her neighborhood, and sometimes her neighbors join in and they visit and talk. She tries to walk 30 minutes almost every day, but sometimes her back is acting up. Then she may walk five to ten minutes several times a day.

When Mama's back is really giving her problems or it's raining, she may do armchair exercises. Her exercise therapist told her about armchair exercise videos she could borrow from the library or buy. Mama likes the seated exercises she does along with the video because she feels more flexible and limber after doing them. If you're interested in armchair exercises, talk with your diabetes health care team to see if seated exercises might be right for you. For more on armchair videos, check with your local library or go online on your computer.

Michael told me he wanted to be more active, but he didn't know what to do since he couldn't play football anymore. I asked Michael to come up with a

list of ideas of things he might want to do. Here's
Michael's list:

- Go to the gym two days a week.
- Play softball with his friends.
- Walk and jog two days a week.

Michael decided to start by walking twice a
week. When the weather is bad, he will go to the
gym. Michael hopes to start walking three times a
week next month.

Get Ready to Be More Active

Take the first step toward making a plan to be more
active. Talk with your diabetes team about what
kinds of activity you think you would like to do.

You might do something that keeps your heart
strong and uses up extra blood sugar and calories,
like swimming, walking, or dancing. You also might
do gentle stretching or strength training to keep
your joints loose and your muscles strong.

If you have diabetes problems, talk with your
diabetes team to find out which exercise choices are
safe for you.

Get Set

When you've built up to longer and more active
workouts, here are a few things to keep in mind:

- Ask your diabetes team about when to check your
  blood sugar. In general, check your blood sugar
  before you exercise. If it's below 100, have a carb

snack that is about 15 grams carbohydrate. This might be a piece of fruit or a handful of pretzels before you start.

- If your fasting blood sugar is above 300, exercise can make your blood sugar go even higher. Talk with your diabetes team about what to do.
- Start slowly to warm up. Stretch your muscles. At the end, slow down to cool off before you stop.
- Stretch again to finish up.
- Attach your medical ID to your shoes or clothing and carry a wallet card.
- Carry a carb food with you. Then you'll be ready to treat low blood sugar if it happens. Glucose tablets, sugar packets, or a small box of raisins are easy to carry.
- Drink plenty of water before, during, and after exercise.

Go for It: Making a Plan and Getting Started

Making a plan will help you reach your goal, step by step. Think of your plan as a deal you make with yourself. Read on to see how Pam and Michael made their plans for adding exercise to their daily routine.

What's my goal for exercise?

Pam's answer: I want to be more active to keep my blood sugar, blood pressure, and blood fats down.

Michael's answer: I want to be more active so I look and feel better.

What's your answer? _____

_____

Why haven't I exercised before?

Pam's answer: I didn't exercise before because I thought I was too busy.

Michael's answer: I couldn't play football anymore. I was sad about that and couldn't get started with anything else.

What's your answer? _____

_____

How can I work around this problem?

Pam's answer: I'll choose activities I can do at home or close to home and that won't take a lot of time.
Michael's answer: I'll talk with my friends about a softball team.

What's your answer? _____

_____

Here's my plan (what I'll do, when, and how long I'll do it):

Pam's answer: I will walk 30 minutes five times a week. I will break this up into two 15-minute sessions or three 10-minute sessions if I'm short on time.

Michael's answer: I will join a summer softball team and play with my friends. This winter I'll walk or go to the gym three days a week.

What's your answer? _____

_____

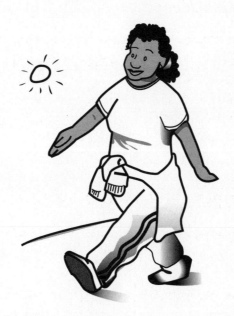

What do I need to get ready?

Pam's answer: I need some new walking shoes that fit well.

Michael's answer: I need to register for the softball team. This winter I'll need to sign up at the gym.

What's your answer? _____

_____

What might get in the way of making this change?

Pam's answer: The weather might not be good.

Michael's answer: The softball game might be rained out.

What's your answer? _____

_____

How can I get around the problem of making a change?

Pam's answer: I'll walk inside or do exercises on TV.

Michael's answer: I'll dance with my girlfriend.

What's your answer? _____

_____

Here's how I'll reward myself:

Pam's answer: If I meet my goals this week, I'll buy myself a flower.

Michael's answer: If I meet my goals this week, I'll go to the movies.

What's your answer? _____

_____

Go for It!

Now that you have your plan, talk it over with your health care team. Do you need a checkup before getting started?

Remember, motion is the potion! Set your start date!

- **My start date for getting up and getting going is** _____

Chapter 11

Guidelines for Diabetes Care

Most people with diabetes need to see their health care provider every three to six months. Before your next diabetes visit, there are things you can do to be sure you're getting up-to-date diabetes care.

Guidelines from the American Diabetes Association can help people with diabetes live long and healthy lives. Called the Standards of Care, these guidelines describe the best diabetes care.

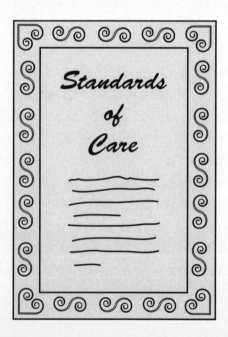

Make sure your health care provider uses the Standards of Care to get the most out of your diabetes visits.

At Every Diabetes Visit

If your diabetes health team is following the Standards of Care, at every diabetes visit your team members will

- **Check your blood pressure.** Your blood pressure numbers tell you the force of blood flow inside your vessels. When your blood pressure is high, your heart has to work harder. If your blood pressure is not on target, work with your diabetes health team. Meal planning, exercise, and medicines can help.
- **Check your weight.** Preventing weight gain or losing weight may be part of your diabetes care plan. If you need to lose weight, even losing 10 to 15 pounds can help you reach your target goals.
- **Answer your questions.** When you think of questions between diabetes visits, write them down. Take your list with you for your next visit. Write down the answers to your questions so that you can review them later.
- **Listen to your concerns.** Are you worried about your kidneys or eyes? Talk with your diabetes team about your concerns and worries.
- **Talk to you about ways to quit smoking, if you smoke**. For more on stopping smoking, see Chapter 16.

At Least Twice a Year

The Standards of Care guidelines suggest that your diabetes care team do this check at least twice a year:

- **Measure your A-1-C level**. This is the blood sugar check with a memory. Your A-1-C reflects your average blood sugar over the last two or three months. It provides the big picture to you and to your diabetes team.

Every Year

The Standards of Care guidelines suggest that your diabetes health care team do these checks at least once a year:

- **Check your cholesterol** (kuh-LES-tuh-rawl) and other blood fats. Your blood cholesterol level may need to be checked more often if you have a problem. See Chapter 19 for more on blood fats and cholesterol.
- **Examine your feet.** Take your shoes and socks off when you go into the exam room. Your provider can check for nerve damage or other problems. Your feet may need to be checked more often if you're having foot problems. Learn more about feet in Chapter 19.
- **Measure your microalbumin** (MY-crow-alb-YOU-min) to check for small amounts of protein in your urine. The microalbumin check tells you how well your kidneys are working. See Chapter 19 for more on the microalbumin check.

- **Refer you to an eye doctor for an eye exam.** Be sure your eye doctor uses eye drops to dilate your eyes so he or she can see the back of your eye. See Chapter 19 for more on eye care.
- **Refer you for diabetes education and nutrition counseling.** You may need a change in your diabetes care plan.
- **Offer you a flu shot.** Every year ask for a flu shot to keep from getting sick.
- **Offer you a pneumonia vaccine.** You need the pneumonia (NEW-moan-ya) vaccine at least once in your lifetime. When you turn 65, you will need another pneumonia vaccine, unless you had one within the last five years.

Mama and her health care team work together using the guidelines from the American Diabetes Association. They talk about her A-1-C results and other lab results. The results help them know how her diabetes care plan is working and about her health.

Things to Do before Each Diabetes Visit

Before each visit with Dr. Wood, Mama does the following things to get the most from her visit:

- **Makes a list of questions.** Dr. Wood and Mama start every visit by going down her list. Questions she sometimes asks are:

  - When is my next A-1-C check?
  - Is my A-1-C target still 6?
  - How is my microalbumin?

- **Makes a list of all of her medicines.** Dr. Wood
  reviews this list with Mama. To make a list of
  your medicines, see the My Medicines form in the
  Diabetes Tools section at the end of this book.
- **Makes a list of her over-the-counter
  medicines.** Some over-the-counter medicines can
  affect your blood pressure and blood sugar.
  Dr. Wood and Mama review this list, too. The
  My Medicines form in the Diabetes Tools section
  at the end of this book also has a section to list
  your over-the-counter medicines.
- **Takes her blood sugar logbook.** Mama and
  Dr. Wood look for patterns in her blood sugars to
  see if her diabetes care plan needs to be changed.
- **Takes paper and pen.** Mama likes to write
  down what Dr. Wood tells her, so she won't forget.
- **Takes a family member with her.** Mama likes
  for me or one of her sisters to go with her for her
  diabetes visit. Mama relies on us for help and
  support.
- **Learns about new diabetes treatments.**
  Mama reads the magazine ***Diabetes Forecast***
  each month. She talks to Dr. Wood about new
  treatments and ways to prevent health problems.
  Mama feels more in charge of her diabetes care
  when she's learning new things about diabetes.

Taking Charge of Your Diabetes Visits

You can get the most out of your diabetes visit by
being prepared. See the list above of things Mama
does for each of her diabetes visits. Also track your
targets. Make a copy of the **Tracking Your**

Targets chart at the end of this chapter to take with you to your diabetes visits. Work with your health care provider to fill in the blanks and to see if you are meeting your goals.

Or you can call the American Diabetes Association toll free at 1-800-DIABETES (800-342-2383) and ask for a copy of the Diabetes Outcomes Card, order code 5984-02. It's a wallet-sized card you can use to record your goals and to track your progress. If your diabetes treatment plan isn't working, talk with your provider about changing your plan. Ask your provider if seeing a diabetes specialist would help.

Tracking Your Targets

The ADA suggests these targets for most people with diabetes. You may have different targets. You can record your targets and your results in the spaces provided here

What to Do	ADA Targets	My Targets	My Results Date	Date
At Every Office Visit				
Review blood sugar numbers				
Before meals	90–130			
2 hours after the start of a meal	Below 180			
Check blood pressure	Below 130/80			
Review meal plan				
Review activity level				
Check weight				
Discuss questions or concerns				
At Least Twice a Year				
A-1-C	Below 7			

Tracking Your Targets *continued*

What to Do	ADA Targets	My Targets	My Results Date	My Results Date
At Least Once a Year				
Physical exam				
Cholesterol				
LDL cholesterol	Below 100			
HDL cholesterol	Above 40 (for men)			
	Above 50 (for women)			
Triglycerides	Below 150			
Dilated eye exam				
Microalbumin	Below 30			
Flu shot				
Once				
Pneumonia vaccine				

Chapter 12

Diabetes Medicines

People with type 2 diabetes will need changes in their diabetes care plan over time. When you first learned you had type 2 diabetes, you may have changed how much or what you ate. You may have started taking walks to keep your blood sugar in your target range. As time goes on, you may need diabetes pills or insulin shots, too. That doesn't mean your diabetes is getting worse. It just means that your old plan isn't working now. Changing your diabetes treatment plan can help you reach your blood sugar goals.

When Mama and Pam were diagnosed with type 2 diabetes, they were able to keep their blood sugar levels in their target range most of the time without taking diabetes medicines. They lost weight, counted their carbs, walked to be more active, and checked their blood sugar with a meter. They worked hard to keep their blood sugar in their target range.

When Nathan found out he had diabetes, changing his food and increasing his activity didn't bring his blood sugar down into his target range. He needed to add a diabetes pill to his treatment plan.

That did the trick, and Nathan's blood sugar levels were back in his target range.

But as time went by, Nathan noticed that his blood sugar wasn't in his target range as often. Nathan's doctor noticed that his A-1-C results were creeping up. Nathan's doctor suggested that Nathan take a second kind of diabetes pill. One kind works during the night. The other works after each meal. Taking two pills doesn't mean that Nathan's diabetes is worse. It just means that the pills work even better together than if he only took one kind without the other. Together the two pills made Nathan feel better, and his blood sugar and A-1-C are back on target.

Different diabetes pills work in different ways to keep blood sugar on track. There are many kinds of diabetes pills, and new ones are on the way. Some people with type 2 diabetes take one kind of pill. Others take two kinds of pills or a combination pill because the drugs work even better together.

What Kind of Pill Is It?

Diabetes pills work in different ways to keep blood sugar on track. When you get your pills, ask the pharmacist what your pills do and if they have any side effects or things to look out for. Put a check next to the kinds of pills you take. Then write down the names of your pills, the amount to take, and when to take them.

☐ **Sulfonylureas** (SUL-fah-nil-YOO-ree-ahz).
They help your body make more insulin.

Name:_____

Amount: _____ How often:_____

When to take: _____

☐ **Biguanides** (by-GWAN-ides). They lower the amount of stored sugar that's released from your liver into your body.

Name:_____

Amount: _____ How often:_____

When to take: _____

☐ **Thiazolidinediones** (THY-ah-ZO-lih-deen-DY-owns). They lower your body's resistance to insulin. This helps your insulin work even better.

Name:_____

Amount: _____ How often:_____

When to take: _____

☐ **Meglitinides** (meh-GLIT-in-ides). They help your body release a quick burst of insulin when you eat a meal or snack.

Name:_____

Amount: _____ How often:_____

When to take: _____

☐ **Alpha-glucosidase inhibitors** (Al-fah gloo-KOHS-ih-dayz in-HIB-it-ers). They slow down the rate at which carbs get into your blood after you eat.

Name:_____

Amount: _____ How often:_____

When to take: _____

☐ **Combination diabetes pills.**

Name:_____

Amount: _____ How often:_____

When to take: _____

☐ **Other pills.**

Name: _____

Amount: _____ How often:_____

When to take: _____

☐ **Other pills.**

Name:_____

Amount: _____ How often:_____

When to take: _____

Don't forget about the My Medicines form in the Diabetes Tools section at the back of the book. You may prefer to use it rather than filling in your medicines above.

Insulin

When Nathan had surgery, his diabetes pills weren't keeping his blood sugar in his target range, so he took insulin shots. He needed shots for several weeks afterwards, too. Nathan said, "I was really scared the first time I gave myself a shot. But it wasn't as bad as I thought it would be. At first I was also worried that once I started taking insulin shots, I'd have to take them forever."

But that's not true. It all depends on what's going on. Sometimes you may need insulin for a short time to keep your blood sugar in your target range.

Nathan used a syringe for his insulin shots, but some people use an insulin pen. An insulin pen has a small needle and a cartridge of insulin that's easy to use.

Some people take both pills and insulin. Robert was having blood sugar readings that were too high in the morning. His team suggested that adding an insulin shot in the evening might help keep his morning blood sugar in his target range. Robert thought it over and decided to try it. He found it was easier to stay in his target range during the day if his blood sugar started out lower in the morning.

If you need to add insulin or if you're using insulin now, here are a few helpful facts about insulin:

- Insulin can't be taken as a pill. Insulin is a protein and would be digested like other protein foods you eat.
- There are different types of insulin:

  - **Rapid-acting** insulins, such as lispro (Humalog), aspart (Novolog), and glulisine (Apidra) are the fastest of all insulins. Once you inject rapid-acting insulin, it starts working within five minutes. It works hardest, or peaks, an hour or so after you inject it. This kind of insulin is designed so you can inject it right before meals. It starts to work about the time you start to eat. By the time your meal is digested and sugar (glucose) is beginning to move into your blood, rapid-acting insulin is working the hardest at moving the blood sugar into your body cells for energy.

- **Short-acting,** or **regular,** insulin is also used around mealtime. It takes longer to work than rapid-acting insulin does. You take short-acting insulin about 30 to 45 minutes before you plan to eat. It peaks about two or three hours later. It can keep working for as long as six hours. Rapid-acting and short-acting insulin are both "clear" in color.

- **Intermediate-acting** insulins, such as NPH and lente, take longer to work. They provide background insulin, but not for meals. They begin to work two to four hours after you inject them. They peak 8 to 14 hours after being injected. They continue to work for 10 to 20 hours. Intermediate-acting insulin works all day if you take it in the morning. It works all night and with morning blood sugars if you take it in the evening. This type of insulin looks "cloudy" and needs to be mixed before injecting.

- **Long-acting** insulins, such as glargine (some-times called Lantus) or ultralente, are usually taken in the morning or at bedtime. Glargine starts to work in about an hour and continues

to work for 24 hours with little or no peak.
Ultralente starts to work 6 to 10 hours after
you inject it and lasts for 18 to 20 hours. Long-
acting insulins can help keep your insulin and
blood sugar levels steady throughout the day
and night.

Insulin Shots

Selecting a syringe

There are different sizes of syringes. Use the size
that is easiest for you to use with your dose of
insulin. Also use a syringe big enough that you can
read the lettering on the side.

Thin, short needles hurt less. If you're
overweight, a short needle may not work for you.
Talk with your diabetes team.

Many people can safely reuse syringes. However,
if you are sick or have open wounds on your hands,
don't risk reusing a syringe. Keep the needle clean
by keeping it capped when not in use. Cleaning the
needle with alcohol will remove the coating that
helps the needle slide into the skin easily. Keep the
needle clean by letting it touch only clean skin and
the top of the insulin bottle.

How to give yourself an insulin shot

If you need to start taking insulin, work with your
diabetes health care team to learn how to do it.
You'll recall that Nathan had to start insulin after

having surgery. He was really scared the first time he gave himself a shot. But it wasn't as bad as he thought it would be.

Here are the basics for giving an insulin shot. If you have questions, ask your diabetes team for help.

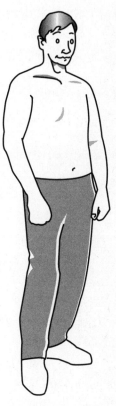

- Decide where to give your insulin shot. You can give your shots pretty much wherever you have enough fat under the skin. The main areas are your stomach, your thighs, and the back of your upper arms. Changing the site where you give your shots is called site rotation. Site rotation prevents a buildup of fat under your skin. Each shot site is about the size of a quarter. You only need to move a finger-width away to give your next shot.

  - Most people prefer to give the shots in their stomach. Your stomach is easy to reach. Also, the insulin is absorbed at a steady rate from shot to shot. If you inject in your stomach, don't get too close to your navel, or belly button. The skin around your navel is tougher and makes the insulin action less smooth.
  - If you inject in your thigh, use the top and outside area. Stay away from your inner thigh.

- ■ If you inject in your arm, use the outer back area of your upper arm. This is where you have the most fat.
- ■ Some people rotate within only one area, like their stomach. Others give their morning shot in their stomachs and their evening shot in their thigh. Talk with your diabetes team about the best options for you.

- ● Wash and dry your hands and wipe the top of the insulin bottle with alcohol.
- ● Before you open the insulin bottle, check the date on it. If it's past that date, don't use it. The insulin is too old.
- ● Check your insulin before using it.

  - ■ Rapid- and short-acting insulins and glargine are clear. If that kind of insulin has changed color, is cloudy, or has little bits in it, it is no good. Throw the bottle away.
  - ■ Intermediate-acting insulin and ultralente are cloudy. If you see any large clumps, throw away the bottle.

- ● If you're using intermediate-acting or ultralente 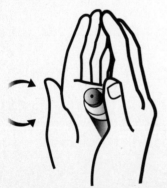 long-acting insulin (cloudy), roll the insulin bottle in your hands gently to mix up the insulin. Don't shake the bottle. Shaking can make the insulin clump. Clear insulins don't need to be rolled.

- If you're injecting both clear and cloudy insulin, check how many units of cloudy insulin you need. Hold the syringe with the needle pointing to the ceiling. Then pull the plunger to that many units on the syringe. You now have a syringe full of air. If you're not using cloudy insulin, go on to the next step about using clear insulin.

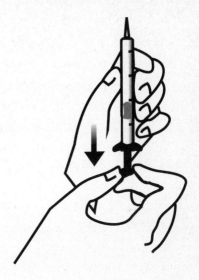

- Put the cloudy insulin bottle on a table or counter and push the needle into the insulin bottle. Don't let the needle touch the insulin. Push in the plunger to put air into the bottle. Now take the needle out of the bottle. The syringe is now empty.

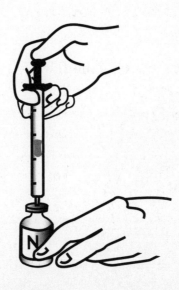

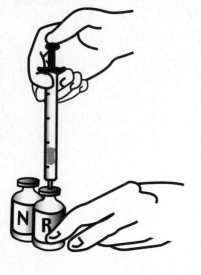

- Check to see how many units of clear insulin you need. Pull back the plunger of the syringe to that number. You now have a syringe with air in it again.
- Put the clear insulin bottle on the table or counter and push the needle into the top. Push the plunger to put air into the bottle. Leave the needle in the bottle.
- Turn the bottle upside down while holding the needle in the bottle. Then pull out the plunger to measure a bit more rapid- or short-acting insulin than you need.
- With the needle still in the upside down bottle, tap the syringe gently. Any air bubbles will rise to the top. Now push the syringe in to get rid of the extra air and the extra insulin.

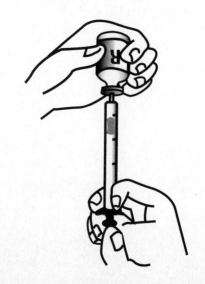

- Check to see that you have the right amount of clear insulin in the syringe. Now take the needle out of the insulin bottle.
- Now it's time to draw up your cloudy insulin. If you only use clear

insulin, skip this step.
Stick the needle in the
top of the intermediate-
acting insulin or ultra-
lente, which are the
cloudy insulins. Turn
the syringe and the
bottle with it upside
down. Now pull out the
plunger slowly to
measure the exact
amount you need. The
exact amount will be

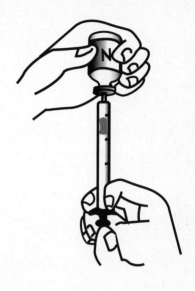

the cloudy insulin plus the clear insulin. Do **not**
push any insulin back into this bottle.

- Double check that you have the right amount of
  insulin. Now pull the needle out of the bottle.
- If you have too much insulin in the syringe, you'll
  need to start over again. If you push the extra
  insulin back into the bottle, you'll be mixing the
  two insulins together in the bottle.
- When you've got the right amount and right kinds
  of insulin in the syringe, it's time to give the shot.
- Pinch an inch of skin where you plan to inject the
  insulin. Pinching an inch makes sure you shoot

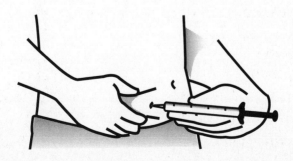

into fat and not into a muscle. Shooting into a muscle hurts more, and it changes how fast the insulin is used by your body.

- Keep pinching with one hand. With the other hand, hold the syringe like a pencil. Look at the needle to see if it's at the right angle. The angle depends on how tough your skin is and other things. Ask your diabetes educator which angle is best for you.
- Gently stick the needle in the skin at the right angle for you. Press the plunger with your thumb gently and steadily until all the insulin is gone. Check to see if injecting the insulin a little slower or a little faster feels better to you. Then stick with that speed.
- Pull the needle out at the same angle you put it in.
- Press your finger on the shot site for a few seconds to keep the insulin from leaking. If you do have leaking, check your blood sugar more often during the day to be sure it's not too high.
- If you do have leaking often, these tips will help:

  - Check the angle of the needle. You may need to straighten the angle a little.
  - Push the plunger more slowly when injecting the insulin.
  - Count to ten after pushing in the plunger before removing the needle.
  - Check the shot site. If it feels lumpy, choose another site.

If you take insulin and you don't feel good, always check your blood sugar.

- **If your blood sugar is low,** first eat something that has about 15 grams of carbohydrate. Glucose tablets, 1/2 cup of regular (not diet) soft drink or fruit juice, or 1 cup of nonfat milk are good choices. Wait 15 minutes, and check your blood sugar again. This is sometimes called the 15-15 rule. If your blood sugar is still too low, eat another 15 grams of carbohydrate and wait 15 more minutes. Keep following this 15-15 rule until your blood sugar is at least above 70. If it's going to be a few hours before your next meal, have a snack with carbohydrate. It could be a piece of whole-wheat bread with peanut butter and jelly.
- **Too much insulin.** If you know you took too much insulin, check your blood sugar every two hours and eat extra carbohydrate if your blood sugar is going too low. If you give yourself too much insulin at night, set your alarm clock and check your blood sugar every two hours during the night.
- **If your blood sugar is too high,** be more active. But if your blood sugar is over 300, activity can make it go even higher. If your blood sugar is often too high, talk with your health care team. Your diabetes plan may need to be updated.
- **Too little insulin.** If you know within an hour that you didn't get enough insulin, give yourself another shot with the rest of the dose. If you don't realize it until later, watch your blood sugar level during the rest of the day. Watch how many carbs you eat and be more active.

Taking care of insulin

Here are things to do when you're using insulin:

- If you know you're going to use up a whole bottle of insulin within a month, you can keep it at room temperature. It will keep for up to a month if it's not too hot—over 86 degrees.
- If you keep insulin in the refrigerator, warm it up before your shot. Cold insulin can make the shot hurt. Draw up the right amount of insulin into the syringe. Then gently roll the syringe between your hands until it feels warm.
- Don't store insulin in the freezer. Insulin clumps up below 36 degrees.
- Don't store insulin in direct sunlight or in the glove box of your car.

What to do with used syringes

- Be careful when you throw away your used syringes so they won't hurt anyone else. Needles can hurt whoever takes out the trash or picks up the garbage. Check to see if your town or state has their own rules for getting rid of used syringes.

Taking Your Medicines

You may take medicines to lower your blood pressure, blood sugar, and blood cholesterol levels.

When you're taking lots of medicines, it can be hard to keep track of all of them. Here are some tips that may help you stay healthy:

- Link your pilltaking to something in your day:
  - Always take your medicine after washing your face or brushing your teeth.
  - If you need to take your medicine with food, take it after eating a meal.
  - Use a pill box with sections for each day of the week. The best way yet!

- Ask your diabetes team or pharmacist these questions about your medicines. Write their answers down on a note card or piece of paper and carry it with you:
  - What are the names of my medicines?
    - Brand name
    - Generic name
  - What's the medicine for?
  - What's the strength of my medicines, such as 25 milligrams? Milligrams are sometimes written as mg.
  - How much do I take for one dose?
  - When should I take it?
    - How many times a day?
    - At what times?
    - On an empty stomach?
    - With food?
    - Do I avoid any foods, medicines, or alcohol when I'm taking it?

- Are there any side effects with this medicine?
- What do I do if I have side effects?
- What if I miss a dose?
- How do I store the medicine?
- How long will the supply last?
- What about refills?

There's a chart on taking your medicines in the Diabetes Tools section at the back of this book. There's also room on the chart for over-the-counter medicines, such as aspirin or cough syrup.

Be sure your health care team is aware of all of the medicines you take. In a paper or plastic bag, bring all your pill bottles, including vitamins and herbal and home remedies, with you when you see your health care team. Or fill in the My Medicines chart in the back of this book and take it with you. Your diabetes team can make sure your medicines all work well together. If you start taking any new pills, they'll check to make sure it's okay to mix them with the pills you're already taking.

Chapter 13

Do You Want to Lose Weight?

Losing weight is one of the best things you can do for your health. Extra weight makes it hard for your insulin to work as well as it could. We all know that losing weight is tough. It takes time and can be a battle. But being overweight is also hard. You may not like the way you look. You may wish you felt better and had more energy. Losing weight can do that for you.

Losing 5 to 15 pounds can change the way you look and feel. Here are things you can look forward to:

- You'll have more energy.
- Your clothes will fit better.
- Your blood sugar will stay closer to your target range.
- You'll reduce your risk of heart disease and stroke.
- Your blood pressure and blood cholesterol levels will go down.
- You may be able to stop taking diabetes pills or insulin or you may only need a smaller dose.

Here are some ways you can lose weight and keep it off, even if you've never done it before.

Ways to Lose Weight

- **Eat less food.**

  - Try the Rate Your Plate method. See Chapter 3 for more information on rating your plate.
  - Eat smaller servings instead of giving up the foods you love.
  - Eat a low-calorie soup or salad before your meal. Studies show that people eat fewer calories if they first have a brothy soup (one with lots of liquid and fewer solids) or a large low-calorie salad before their main meal.
  - Use a small plate instead of a large dinner plate. This makes it look like we're getting more food.
  - Serve smaller portions because we tend to eat everything that we're served. When people are served smaller portions, they eat those portions and feel full.
  - Be the last in line at a family gathering. You'll still have food to eat after others have finished eating.
  - Eat more slowly, so you're the last one to finish eating. Cut small bites, chew slowly, and chew well. Putting your fork down between bites also helps. Sipping water between bites slows down eating, too.
  - Have a fruit or vegetable every time you have a meal or snack. This helps fill you up.

- Go for more salad, vegetables, or fruit if you need a second serving.
- Write down what and how much you eat and drink. This helps with eating less because you can see what you're actually eating.
- Order the smallest size when eating out.
- Split entrees and desserts with friends and family when eating out. You'll eat less, and you'll save money, too. Or take some home for later or tomorrow's lunch.
- Buy single-serving sizes of snacks, like chips, instead of big bags. You won't be so tempted to eat more than you planned.
- Make your own snack packs by putting pretzels in a small bag.
- Check serving sizes on food labels. Compare them to the serving sizes you're eating. Often, a can or box has two to four servings in it, so you could be getting two to four times as many carbs as you think.

Can you think of other ways to eat less food?

- _____

- _____

Choose one way to eat less food that you think will work for you and write it here:

_____

   If you can eat less food, you'll begin to lose weight, lower your blood sugar, have more energy, and feel good about yourself.

● **Eat less fat.**

■ Cook lower-fat versions of your favorite recipes.
■ Use fats in small amounts. All fats have lots of calories, even the healthier fats like olive and canola oil, nuts, and seeds.
■ Use nonstick pans and cooking sprays.
■ Use low-fat versions of foods you like, such as cottage cheese, cream cheese, cheese, salad dressings, mayonnaise, margarine, and sour cream. These foods contain saturated fat, which is not good for your blood vessels and heart.
■ Bake, broil, grill, microwave, or roast meats, chicken, and fish.
■ Eat fried or high-fat foods only once or twice a week.
■ Take the skin off chicken and turkey. Eat breasts and drumsticks more often than wings or thighs.
■ Trim the fat off meats.
■ Buy tuna canned in water instead of oil.
■ Try mustard on a sandwich instead of mayonnaise. Or use light mayonnaise.
■ Drink fat-free or low-fat milk instead of whole milk.

Can you think of other ways to eat less fat?

■ _____

■ _____

Choose one way to eat less fat that you think will work for you and write it here:

_____

If you can eat less fat, you'll begin to lose weight, lower your blood sugar, have more energy, and feel better about yourself. You will also have less fat in your blood.

- **Eat regular meals.**

  - Eat some food for breakfast or within a few hours of getting up every day.
  - Eat meals on time. Skipping meals can make you hungrier and moody and lead to eating more at your next meal. Also, if you take diabetes medicines, skipping meals can cause problems.
  - Find the right eating pattern for you. Some people like three meals a day. Others like three meals and a snack. Some eat six small meals a day. Learn what works best for you.
  - Plan ahead what you're going to eat. Be sure you have everything on hand that you'll need. Then when you come in late, you'll already know what you're having for dinner.
  - Prepare some foods ahead of time. You can cook extra meals on the weekend, first thing in the morning, or the night before. Use a crock pot or a pressure cooker to help you have healthier meals in a short time.
  - Try to eat about the same time each day.

    ○ My usual meal times are:

    _____

    ○ My usual snack times are:

    _____

Can you think of other ways to eat regular meals?

■ _____

■ _____

Choose one way to try to eat regular meals that you think will work for you and write it here:

_____

If you can eat regular meals, you'll begin to lose weight, lower your blood sugar and blood cholesterol levels, have more energy, and feel better about yourself.

● **Eat fewer sweets and desserts.**

■ Buy fewer sweets.
■ Buy smaller sized packages.
■ Share a dessert. Try savoring just three bites of a dessert.
■ Drink sugar-free drinks, such as soft drinks and iced tea.
■ Use a low-calorie sweetener on your cereal, in your coffee, and in cooking, instead of sugar.
■ Buy small juice glasses so you'll drink less juice.
■ Mix juice and seltzer water and pour over ice for a juice cooler.
■ Eat a piece of fruit instead of candy.
■ Try sugar-free popsicles if you think you can eat just one at a time.

Can you think of other ways to eat fewer sweets that will work for you?

■ _____

■ _____

Choose one way to eat fewer sweets and desserts that you think will work for you and write it here:

_____

If you can eat fewer sweets, you'll begin to lose weight, lower your blood sugar, have more energy, and feel better about yourself.

Nathan lost 10 pounds and has kept it off for two years. Nathan said, "Losing weight wasn't the hard part for me. In fact, I've lost the same 10 pounds a dozen times, but every time I put it all back on plus a few more pounds.

"Even though it was harder for me to lose weight because of my diabetes medicines, I focused on what I could eat. I didn't focus on 'don't eat this' and 'don't eat that.' I still included the foods I love. I just had smaller portions, except for fruits and vegetables. I practiced portion power. I told myself I could have the other half of whatever it was the next day.

"I eat most of the same foods I always did, but I learned to cut back on fat by not frying, using less fat in recipes, and buying low-fat dairy products and salad dressings. I even have low-fat recipes for oven-fried chicken and mashed potatoes made with fat-free buttermilk.

"I also use a smaller plate, and my servings look bigger. This really helps with my portion power. I try to drink plenty of water and sugar-free drinks, like iced tea.

"Writing down what I eat and how much I walk every day really helps me stay on track. I reward myself each week by going to a ball game. I have great support from my family, friends, and coworkers.

"I've been able to keep the weight off with a plan and some help. If I can do it, everybody can do it."

Knowing When You're Ready to Lose Weight

When you can put a check next to most of the items below, you're ready to lose weight.

- I've thought about why I want to lose weight.
- I think I can do it. I want to do it.
- I've made a plan for changing the way I eat.
- I've made a plan for being more active nearly every day.
- I've thought about how to get around things that have gotten in my way before.
- I've asked my family, friends, and coworkers for support.
- I've talked with my health care team about my plan, and I've gotten the help I need from them.

Making Your Plan to Lose Weight

If you're ready to lose weight, these questions will help you make your plan:

- Why do I want to lose weight?

  _____

- What's hard about losing weight for me?

  _____

- How can I work around these problems?

  _____

- Who will help me?

  _____

- What's my plan for losing weight?

  _____

- What's my first step?

  _____

- What do I need to get ready?

  _____

- How will I reward myself?

  _____

- I'll start my plan on _____ (date).

- My weight loss goal is to lose ____ pounds in one month. (I suggest to most of the people I work with to try for two to four pounds per month.)

- My weight loss goal is to lose ____ pounds in six months.

- My weight loss goal is to lose ____ pounds in the next year.

How to Track Your Progress

There are many ways to track your success. Choose one or more ways that will be helpful to you.

- Write down what you eat and drink.
- Write down when you eat. If you eat but you're not hungry, write down why you're eating, too.
- Write down the amount of activity you've done. This can be as simple as a hatch mark for

$\cancel{||||} \; || = 70$ minutes
of walking

    10 minutes of walking. Add up the hatch marks at the end of the week to see how you're doing.

- Weigh yourself once a week or once a month. It doesn't matter which one. Keep a log of your weight over time. This will let you see if your plan is working. The best time to check your weight is the first thing in the morning, before you eat or drink anything.
- Use your clothes to measure your success. Can you tighten to the next hole on your belt? Are your jeans fitting better? Can you wear a shirt you haven't worn for awhile?

    Don't be tempted by promises of quick weight loss. Watch out for programs that promise you can eat all that you want and still be able to lose weight. Don't be fooled by programs that claim to be easy, quick, or new or that will melt fat away.

    Tried and true weight loss methods help you form new habits to lose weight and keep you going until you reach your goal weight. And then those habits will help you keep the weight off that you lost.

Chapter 14

Diabetes and Depression

It's hard to hear that you have type 2 diabetes or pre-diabetes. It's also hard to live with diabetes on a daily basis. There's never a break from diabetes. There's never a vacation from diabetes. Caring for your diabetes takes time and effort. Sometimes the burden of diabetes can seem like too much to handle. Feeling sad and blue and depressed at times is common for everybody. But if you feel down for two weeks or more, talk with your diabetes health care team. You may have depression.

Diabetes doubles the risk for depression. Depression occurs in one of every three people with diabetes. Serious depression is a medical problem, like having high blood pressure or high cholesterol. This is nothing to feel ashamed about. **The good news is that there are treatments that can help.**

If you have serious depression, it can be hard to get out of bed, do your work, or enjoy anything. You might have trouble being with family and friends or taking care of your diabetes. Counseling or medicine can help you feel better. You'll be able to start enjoying life again. And you'll be able to take care of your diabetes.

Nathan was really down for a few weeks last spring. Spring is his best time of year, but Nathan wasn't able to enjoy the warmer weather or working in his garden. He couldn't focus on taking care of his diabetes. Nathan felt so down that he didn't bother to check his blood sugar. He didn't care if his blood sugar was out of his target range.

Nathan ran into a friend who also has diabetes. She said, "Nathan, you don't look so good. Is there anything wrong?" Nathan said he was feeling really down. She said, "Nobody likes to talk about feeling down. They worry that people will think they're weak if they admit they're depressed."

Nathan talked with some of his friends, but it wasn't enough. He talked with his diabetes educator about feeling down and not taking care of his diabetes. Nathan's diabetes educator suggested that he see a therapist.

Over time, talking with the therapist and taking medicine helped Nathan. He told his friends, "Get help if you feel depressed for two weeks or more. If you aren't enjoying your hobbies or can't do your work or go to school, get help."

Nathan said, "At first I thought that feeling down was my own fault. But I learned that when you have diabetes, you may have physical changes that can lead to depression. Counseling and medicine helped me a lot. I'm glad I got help.

"My depression is gone, and I'm enjoying gardening again. I'm taking care of my diabetes and going to work every day. But I know that because I have diabetes, it could come back. I also know what to do if it does. I'll get help a lot sooner."

Signs of Depression

Watch out for signs that you might need help. Talk with your health care team about help if these things describe you:

- You've been feeling low or depressed for two weeks or more.
- You've lost interest in things that used to be fun.
- You've gained or lost a lot of weight.
- You're eating more than usual.
- You're eating less than usual.
- You're unable to sleep.
- You're sleeping too much.
- You're unable to make decisions.
- You're having trouble focusing or thinking things through.
- You feel tired and don't have any energy.

Sometimes it helps to have the support of family and friends. Mama felt sad when she learned she had diabetes. It made her feel down. She didn't like it. Luckily, her family was there to help. She didn't have to go through it alone. Neither do you.

Talk with your friends and family about how you feel and what they can do to help. Maybe you need someone to go with you while you walk. Or maybe you need someone to go with you to your diabetes classes or to your visits with your health care team. But family and friends may not be enough. You may need to talk with members of your health care team, such as the diabetes educator or a counselor.

Living with diabetes isn't easy. While it's normal to be upset sometimes, you don't want these feelings to take over. Here are some tips for coping:

- Write down a list of questions or worries to talk over with your health care team.
- Ask your family and others to support your diabetes care efforts.
- Join a support group.
- Learn more about diabetes, so you can feel in charge and secure.
- Set goals for your diabetes care that you can reach.
- Reach your goals by changing what you do one step at a time.
- Keep in mind that any steps you take toward your goals will help.
- Talk with a therapist if feelings of depression take over your life.
- Being active can also help you feel better when you're depressed. Walking, playing with the kids, dancing, or swimming will help lift your spirits.

If you think you are depressed, get help right away. The sooner you get treatment, the sooner you'll feel better.

Chapter 15

Stress and Diabetes

You know that food, exercise, and diabetes medicines all affect your blood sugar levels. But did you know that stress can make your blood sugar levels go up?

We feel stressed when problems at home or work put us in a strain. Even happy events like taking a trip or your son's wedding can feel stressful. Stress makes it hard to keep your blood sugar on track for two reasons:

- When you're feeling stressed, your body makes hormones that can affect your blood sugar.
- When you're stressed about things in your life, it's hard to take care of your diabetes.

You can't get rid of all the stress in your life, but you can learn to cope with things you can't change.

Mama called me recently saying, "My blood sugar was 275 two hours after my dinner! It's never been that high before. I only had my usual three carb choices at dinner tonight. Do you think my meal plan isn't working anymore?"

We talked about what she had eaten for dinner:

- **1/2 cup black bean and corn salsa**
- **One corn tortilla**
- Grilled chicken breast
- Tossed salad with light salad dressing
- Iced tea
- **1/2 cup sugar-free pudding**

Indeed, Mama had eaten her three carb choices, which are in **bold print** above. I asked her if she felt like she was getting sick with a cold or a sore throat. She said no. Then I asked her if she was worried or stressed about anything.

"Why, yes!" she said. "I was driving today, and a woman in another car started following me and yelling at me. It made me really mad, but it also scared me. It's been on my mind all day. Why would she have done that to me?"

I explained to Mama that her blood sugar was up because the woman upset her and raised her hormones. And those hormones raised her blood sugar. I suggested that Mama check her blood sugar after dinner the next night.

The next night Mama called and was thrilled. Her blood sugar was back in her target range. Mama said, "I guess my meal plan is still working. My blood sugar was high last night because I was stressed."

When Nathan found out he had diabetes, things were tough for him. He wanted to make changes to take care of his diabetes.

"There's so much to learn and take care of," Nathan said. "I feel stressed. I don't even want to be with my family or friends anymore."

Nathan talked with his health care team about feeling stressed. He also told them his blood sugars were high, and he didn't feel good. He was tired all the time. Nathan wanted to get some ideas about what might help.

Nathan's team suggested he go to a diabetes support group. Nathan decided to go. At his first meeting, Nathan felt out of place. But then someone talked about how hard it was for him when he first got diabetes.

"It helped me a lot to know that he had been stressed too," Nathan said. "After a couple of meetings, I didn't feel so alone anymore. The people in the group knew what I was going through. I get a lot of help from them. And I've learned that when I help others, it helps me too."

Are You Stressed Out?

How do **you** feel when you're stressed out? Put a check mark next to the things that are true for you when you're feeling stressed.

- ☐ I get headaches, backaches, or other aches and pains.
- ☐ My muscles get tense.
- ☐ I feel all sweaty.
- ☐ My heart pounds, and I breathe faster.
- ☐ I feel shaky and nervous.
- ☐ I can't sleep.
- ☐ I feel sad.
- ☐ I _____.

Feeling shaky or nervous, breathing fast, or having a fast heartbeat can also be caused by low blood sugar.

What do **you** do when you feel stressed?

- I eat too much.
- I don't feel like eating.
- I drink too much alcohol.
- I smoke a lot.
- I sleep a lot.
- I have trouble sleeping.
- I have trouble remembering things.
- I have a hard time making decisions.
- I lose my temper.
- I worry about everything.
- I don't feel like doing anything.
- I pray and meditate.
- I get cranky.
- I talk to others.
- I _____.

You can't get rid of all the stresses in your life, but you can learn to deal with them. When something goes wrong, don't be hard on yourself. Say to yourself, "I'll do better next time." Set goals that you can reach and feel good about.

Set aside time to relax each day and do something you enjoy. Hobbies, for example, give you time away from daily stresses. Exercise is another way to cope with stress, like taking a yoga class or walking around your neighborhood. Try other new ways to relax. Listening to music, praying, deep breathing, or meditating may help. Also learn to say "no" to things you don't need or don't have to do. Some people can relax by taking a bubble bath, lighting a candle and watching it burn, reading, or listening to the rain.

Chapter 16

Smoking and Diabetes

You know that having diabetes means you're at risk for certain health problems. But smoking increases your risk even higher for heart disease and eye, kidney, and nerve damage. When you have diabetes and you smoke, it means double trouble. Quitting smoking is one of the hardest things you'll ever do, but you'll be glad you did it. It's truly worth the effort.

Double Trouble

What do diabetes and smoking have in common? They put you at risk for many of the same health problems. Consider the top benefits of giving up smoking:

1. Your blood pressure will go down.
2. You're less likely to have

   - foot problems
   - a stroke
   - a heart attack
   - a nerve disease
   - kidney problems

3. Your hair and clothes will smell better.
4. You'll get fewer wrinkles in your face.
5. You'll have healthier gums and teeth.
6. Your loved ones and friends won't be breathing your smoke.
7. You won't have smoker's breath.
8. Your risk for cancer will go down.
9. You'll have more money to spend on other things.
10. If you're a woman, you'll be less likely to have a miscarriage or a stillbirth.
11. If you're a man, you'll be less likely to have erectile dysfunction, also called impotence.

Have you ever tried to quit smoking? It's hard because smoking is addictive. Your body comes to depend on nicotine. And your mind gets addicted, too. There are lots of hurdles to get over as you try to quit smoking.

Nicotine patches, gum, and new medicines can help. Making a plan can also help.

Are You Ready to Quit Smoking?

Before you quit smoking:

- Think of your reasons to stop and write them down. Keep your list where you'll see it every day.
- Tell others you'll need their help and understanding.
- Throw away your cigarettes, lighters, and ashtrays.
- Ask a friend or family member to quit smoking with you.

- Join a stop-smoking group.

If you think you're ready to quit, decide how you'll do it:

- Go cold turkey. Quitting all at once works for some people.
- Quit smoking slowly by cutting back over a few weeks.
- Use a nicotine patch or gum.
- Ask your doctor about new medicines for quitting smoking.

Making a Plan

Robert was sick with a cold and sore throat. His smoking made his sore throat and cough worse. He decided he'd had enough. He wanted to try to quit smoking.

His diabetes team helped him make a plan by answering the questions below. Robert's plan worked for him. Answering these questions will help you make a plan and take the first step toward quitting smoking.

Why do I want to quit smoking?

Robert's answer: I know smoking means big trouble for people with diabetes.

Your answer: _____

_____

Why haven't I quit smoking before?

Robert's answer: Everyone I know smokes.

Your answer: _____

_____

What stopped me from quitting smoking before?

Robert's answer: Smoking helps me handle
stress.

Your answer: _____

_____

I've tried to quit smoking before. Why did I start smoking again?

Robert's answer: The addiction was just too
strong.

Your answer: _____

_____

What can I do to keep from starting again this time?

Robert's answer: I'll use a nicotine patch to help
with the addiction.

Your answer: _____

_____

Who will help me?

Robert's answer: I'll join a support group to learn about other ways to handle stress.

Your answer: _____

_____

What steps will I take to quit smoking?

Robert's answer: I'll hang out with people at work who don't smoke.

Your answer: _____

_____

What do I need to do to quit smoking?

Robert's answer: I'll throw away my cigarettes, lighter, and ashtrays. I'll also ask my wife to quit with me. She said she would try to quit, too.

Your answer: _____

_____

When will be the hardest times?

Robert's answer: My hardest times will be when I'm stressed or when I'm around people who are smoking.

Your answer: _____

_____

What will I do?

Robert's answer: I'll learn other ways to handle stress in the support group. I'll also tell my friends I'm trying to quit and need their help.

Your answer: _____

_____

How will I cope with stress without smoking?

Robert's answer: I'll take short walks to get rid of my stress. It works for me.

Your answer: _____

_____

How will I try to keep from gaining weight?

Robert's answer: I've talked with my diabetes health care team about exercise and meal planning. My wife and I will take walks after dinner most days of the week. This will help both of us.

Your answer: _____

_____

How will I set a date to quit?

Robert's answer: My wife and I have picked a date—July 4th—to be free from cigarettes.

Your answer: _____ (date)

How will I reward myself?

Robert's answer: My wife and I will go on a trip. We will be able to afford it. We won't be spending $8 a day on cigarettes anymore!

Your answer: _____

_____

   "In the past," Robert said, "I wasn't ready to quit. This time I thought about it, made a plan, got help, and set the date. It was hard to do, but I did it. It also helped that my wife quit with me. Having a no-smoking buddy really helps.

   "To keep from smoking now," he said, "I've changed some of my routines. Now I take a short walk after lunch instead of smoking. Quitting smoking was one of the hardest things I've ever done, but I'm glad I did it. I'll do whatever it takes to stay away from smoking."

Chapter 17

Sex and Diabetes

Sex is an important part of life and partnerships. But diabetes can affect your sex life. Problems with having sex are not a normal part of getting older and don't happen to all people with diabetes. There is hope. Talk with your health care team about treatments.

For Men Only

Some men with diabetes have impotence, also called erectile dysfunction or ED (EE-DEE). ED is when a man can no longer have or keep an erection. Over time, blood vessels and nerves in the penis can become damaged. This can lead to ED.

If you have ED, there is hope. There are ways to treat ED that can help. ED is not a normal part of getting older, and it doesn't happen to all men with diabetes. ED can have other causes, such as smoking or prostate or bladder surgery.

It's normal to feel upset if you have ED or some other sexual problem. You may blame yourself or your partner. Some men feel guilty and angry. Others feel like there's no hope. These feelings can make it hard to talk openly with your partner or your doctor. But talking about ED means you're one step closer to getting help.

- There are many ways to treat ED and more are on the way. If one thing doesn't work, something else might. Take with your health care provider about your options, such as taking pills to treat ED. If that doesn't work, there are other treatment options.
- Talk with your doctor to see if any medicines you're taking could be causing ED. Some pills for high blood pressure or for depression may cause ED. Pills for stomach ulcers or heartburn also may cause it. Talk with your doctor before stopping any of your medicines.
- Diabetes raises your risk for depression. Depression can lead to ED, and ED can cause men to feel depressed. Talk with your health care team if you feel depressed. Medicines or counseling can help with depression.

If you have ED, it's not the end of your sex life. It can be hard to talk about ED. Even if your doctor doesn't ask about ED, talk about it if you're having problems. Talking about ED is the only way to learn about treatments and get help.

For Women Only

Some women with diabetes have less interest in sex because of depression or frequent yeast infections. High blood sugar levels can make some women feel tired all of the time. Or perhaps intercourse is painful because of vaginal dryness.

If you find you don't enjoy sex anymore, it's normal to feel upset. You may blame yourself or your partner. Some women feel angry or depressed. These feelings can make it hard for you to talk openly with your partner. Don't give up.

Both depression and anxiety can take away your desire for sex. Medicine or counseling can help with both depression and anxiety. If you're feeling depressed or worried for more than two weeks, talk with your health care team.

What about hormones? Some women find it hard to keep their blood sugar on track the week before and during their menstrual period. Your blood sugar levels may go up or down because of changes in your hormone levels.

Make a note of the days when you're having your period in your blood sugar logbook. Then look for patterns. Is your blood sugar always high during these days? Talk with your health care team about changing your care plan before, during, or after your period to keep your blood sugar levels on target.

Menopause (MEN-oh-paws), also called the change of life, can affect your blood sugar. As your hormone levels change, you may also have hot flashes or other signs. Talk with your health care team about options. You may need a change in your diabetes plan because changes in hormone levels can affect blood sugar. Also, some women gain weight during menopause. Changing your meal plan or being more active can help keep your weight where you want it.

Here's a list of things you may want to talk about with your health care team. Find a member of your team you feel comfortable with. Take a list like this with you to your next diabetes visit:

- Sex is painful for me.
- I don't enjoy sex as much as I did before.
- I'm less interested in sex than before.
- I often have yeast infections.
- I have irregular periods.
- I often feel very sad for more than two weeks.
- I often feel very worried.
- I don't feel like I can cope.
- It's hard to stay in my blood sugar target range before or during my period.
- I'm going through the change of life. I would like to know about my options.

Pregnancy and Diabetes

Are you and your partner thinking about having a baby? Diabetes doesn't affect your ability to become a father or a mother. Talk with your health care team if you have questions or concerns.

For women with diabetes who are thinking about becoming pregnant, start working with your health care team well before you get pregnant. Have your A-1-C, blood pressure, heart, kidneys, nerves, and eyes checked. See your dietitian to review your meal plan. Talk with your team about how being pregnant will affect your long-term health. If you take diabetes pills, you may need to switch to insulin to protect your baby. You may be referred to a special diabetes and pregnancy team.

You will keep yourself and your baby healthy and safe if you keep your blood sugar in your target range before you get pregnant and until the baby arrives. That will lower your chances of having a premature baby or a baby that's larger than normal. You'll also lower the risk of having a baby with birth defects by keeping your blood sugar close to normal in the first weeks of pregnancy.

Today, more women with diabetes are able to have healthy babies. With planning and hard work, you can too.

Birth Control and Diabetes

If you don't want to get pregnant, you'll need to use some kind of birth control. Even if you don't have regular periods, you can still get pregnant. Most birth control methods are safe for women with diabetes. Talk with your health care team about birth control options.

Chapter 18

Alcohol and Diabetes

If you have type 2 diabetes, you may wonder about drinking alcohol. Alcohol can lower or raise your blood sugar. That sounds confusing. The effect of alcohol on blood sugar depends on how much alcohol you drink and if you drink the alcohol with food.

Guidelines for Drinking Alcohol with Type 2 Diabetes

For people with type 2 diabetes, here are some guidelines for drinking alcohol safely:

- Discuss drinking alcohol with your diabetes health care team.
- Drink alcohol only if your blood sugar levels are in your target range most of the time.
- Limit alcohol to one drink a day if you're a woman and to two drinks a day if you're a man.

  - One drink is equal to

    - 12 ounces of beer
    - 5 ounces of wine

○ 1 1/2 ounces of distilled spirits, such as scotch or bourbon.

- Always drink alcohol with a meal or snack that contains carbohydrates. Treat alcohol as an addition to your meal or snack. No food needs to be skipped.
- Alcohol makes it harder to know if you have low blood sugar. Drink with a friend or someone who knows you have diabetes and who can treat low blood sugar.
- Mix alcohol with water, club soda, seltzer, or diet drinks. Try a wine spritzer that is made with club soda rather than a wine cooler.
- Stay away from sweet wines, liqueurs, and sweet mixed drinks, such as a margarita.
- Avoid alcohol if you're pregnant or if you've abused alcohol in the past.
- Avoid alcohol if you have other medical problems. Alcohol can make some problems worse.

Robert went out for a beer with his friends after work on a Friday night. There weren't any pretzels on the table like there usually were. They were having a good time and ordered a second round of beers. Tom, one of Robert's friends, noticed that Robert was starting to sweat and seemed confused. Tom said, "Robert, I think your blood sugar is low. Let's all order some sandwiches." After eating the sandwich, Robert felt better.

Robert said, "Thanks, Tom! I needed your help. My blood sugar was low, and I think the beers made it hard for me to know it."

Chapter 19

Long-Term Diabetes Problems

You may be worried about getting long-term diabetes problems, called diabetes complications. Mama was worried about diabetes problems when she found out she had diabetes. She knew all about diabetes problems from her sister, Carla. My patient Michael worried about diabetes problems, too. He knew about the problems his grandparents had from diabetes. Lots of people with diabetes feel this way.

But the good news is that you can put off or prevent diabetes problems. The key actions you can take right now to protect yourself from diabetes problems are

- Keep blood sugar, blood pressure, and blood fats in your target range. Studies have shown time and again how important this is.
- If you smoke, ask your health care team for help with quitting.
- Stay in contact with your diabetes health care team so that any problems can be found early and treated.

Now let's look at the problems of diabetes one at a time.

Eyes

People with diabetes can have eye problems, also called retinopathy (reh-tih-NOP-uh-thee). Carlos is sad about losing his eyesight from type 2 diabetes. Carlos says, "Do what your health care team tells you. I wouldn't be blind if I had taken care of my diabetes. I wish I had a second chance. I'd work with my diabetes team and take care of my diabetes."

At first there may not be any warning signs of diabetes eye problems. Later on, there may be changes in your eyesight, such as double vision, floating spots, or flashing lights, or you may have trouble seeing.

But you can delay or prevent eye problems by having an eye exam every year. Be sure your

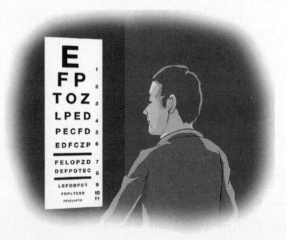

eye doctor uses eye drops to dilate your eyes. By dilating your eyes, the doctor can see the back of your eye and check for problems. Also try to keep your blood sugar and blood pressure in your target range to protect your eyes.

If you have an eye problem, your vision might be affected forever if you don't get treated. There are ways to treat diabetic eye problems. Most blindness in people with diabetes can be prevented if it is treated early. Your doctor can use laser therapy to help protect your eyes if you have a problem. A beam of light is aimed through the pupil of your eye to seal weak places in the small blood vessels of your eye.

If you've just been told you have type 2 diabetes, talk to your health care team about referring you to an eye doctor right away. Then have an eye exam every year. Your eyesight is worth it.

Feet

Bill worked in retail and sold shoes. He spent a lot of time on his feet. By the end of the day, his feet would get really tired. Bill said, "Then I got a problem. Even when my feet should have been hurting, I didn't feel a thing. I needed the pain to tell me when I had a problem. But after 20 years with diabetes, my feet didn't feel pain, heat, or cold.

"During a shoe sale at the store, I bought a new pair of shoes and wore them all day. I got a blister but didn't feel it. Before I noticed, the blister had turned into a nasty ulcer.

"One morning after my shower, I saw the ulcer. I went to the doctor right away. I had to go to the hospital for a few days and take antibiotics.

"If I'd let that ulcer go untreated, I might have lost my foot. That's what happened to my Uncle Mike. That's really scary. Now I check my feet every night, no matter what."

After people have had type 2 diabetes over time, they may have less blood flow to their feet and legs. Minor problems can become big problems and take longer to heal.

Here are some things you can do to protect your feet:

- Keep your blood sugar levels in your target range most of the time. High blood sugar over time can damage the blood vessels and the nerves that go to your feet.
- Check your feet every day. You might want to check your feet after your bath or shower or when you're getting dressed. Look at the tops, bottoms, sides, and between the toes. Use a mirror if you can't see the bottoms or sides of your feet. Or ask someone to check your feet for you. Watch for

  - Blisters, cuts, redness, swelling, sores, or breaks in your skin.
  - Corns and calluses. If you have corns or calluses, gently use a pumice stone each day. Don't cut corns or calluses. This can lead to an infection. Also avoid corn removers, but you can use a pad to relieve pressure until the corn heals.
  - Ingrown toenails or toenail infections.

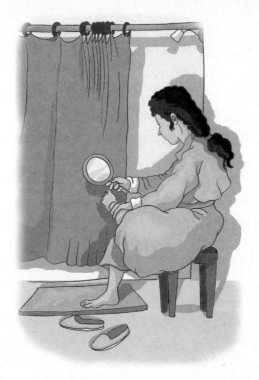

- ■ Feel your feet for cold or hot spots, bumps, or dry skin.

- Wash your feet with warm water and mild soap. Check the water with your wrist first so you won't burn your feet.
- Dry your feet well. Be sure to dry between your toes.
- Use lotion if your skin is dry. Don't use lotion between your toes. Infections can grow in dark moist places.
- Trim or file your nails to match the shape of your toes. Rounded edges help prevent ingrown toenails. If you aren't able to trim your nails, ask someone for help. Your diabetes educator, doctor,

or a podiatrist (foot doctor) can help with foot care.

- Never walk barefoot anywhere, and be careful about wearing sandals.
- Check inside your shoes to be sure there are no objects, like a small stone.
- Protect your feet from hot or cold. Wear shoes at the beach or on hot surfaces. Don't use heating pads or hot water bottles. You can burn your feet without knowing it.

Your diabetes health care team can help you prevent foot problems. At every diabetes visit, remind them to look at your feet by taking off your shoes and socks. Ask your provider for a complete foot exam at least once a year, and more often if you have a foot problem.

One way to check the feeling in your feet is with a monofilament (mahn-oh-FILL-a-ment). It looks like a piece of nylon fishing line or a bristle in a brush. Then you and your provider will know if you have areas that are numb in your feet.

Your provider will look at your skin to check for injuries and may do other foot checks such as pulses and reflexes. He'll check for changes in the shape of your foot and look at your toenails.

Most of the time, special shoes and socks aren't needed. If you have nerve damage in your feet, your insurance may pay for special shoes if you need them. Choose socks without bulky seams at the toes and that aren't too tight at the top.

Bill loves shoes! He sells them, and he likes to wear stylish shoes. He looks for the same things in

the shoes he sells as he does in the shoes he buys
for himself:

- Style and good fit to prevent blisters or corns. A
  shoe needs to be long enough to allow the toes to
  wiggle.
- Low-heeled shoes that feel good. High heels put
  too much stress on your feet.
- Insides that don't have any rough edges that
  might rub your feet.

Feet keep us moving and enjoying life. Take care
of yours every day. You want them to last a lifetime.

Heart and Blood Vessels

People with diabetes are more likely to have a heart
attack or stroke. Their heart attacks can be more
serious and can happen early in life to both women
and men.

Heart disease happens when blood vessels
narrow from a buildup of fat. All blood vessels can
be affected. If this happens to the blood vessels to
the heart, it can lead to a heart attack. If the
vessels to the brain are affected, it can lead to a
stroke. If the blood vessels to the legs and feet are
affected, it can lead to peripheral (puh-RIF-uh-rul)
arterial (ar-TEER-ree-ul) disease or PAD. PAD
results in less blood flow to the legs and feet.

**The good news is that you can take steps to
lower your risk for heart attack, stroke, or
PAD**. Making wise food choices, being active, and
taking medicines, if you need them, can lower your

risk and keep your ABCs of diabetes in your target range. So, what are your ABCs of diabetes?

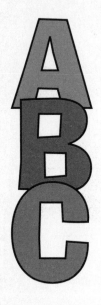

A is for A-1-C. You'll recall that the A-1-C is the blood sugar check with a memory. It tells you your average blood sugar level for the past two to three months. (See Chapter 7 for more on the A-1-C check.)

The American Diabetes Association target for the A-1-C is below 7. But your diabetes health care team may set a different target for you. Keep track of your A-1-C results by using the chart below.

A-1-C

Diabetes Visit	My Results	My Target
Date:		
Date:		
Date:		
Date:		

The American Diabetes Association A-1-C target is below 7.

B is for blood pressure. Your blood pressure is always read as two numbers, such as 130/80, and it's spoken as 130 over 80. The first number is the amount of pressure against your blood vessel walls as your heart beats and pushes blood through the blood vessels. The second number is the pressure when your heart rests between beats. High blood pressure raises your risk for heart attack and stroke.

The American Diabetes Association target for blood pressure is below 130 over 80. Your diabetes health care team may set a different blood pressure target for you. Keep track of your blood results by using the chart below.

Blood Pressure

Diabetes Visit	My Results	My Target
Date:		
Date:		
Date:		
Date:		

The American Diabetes Association blood pressure target is below 130 over 80.

C is for cholesterol. Your cholesterol numbers tell you the amount of fats in your blood. There are different kinds of fat in your blood:

- **LDL cholesterol** is sometimes called the bad cholesterol. It can narrow or block blood vessels. Keeping your LDL cholesterol **low** reduces your risk for heart disease.

  The American Diabetes Association target for LDL cholesterol is below 100. Your diabetes health care team may set a different goal for you. Keep track of your results by using the chart on the next page.

LDL Cholesterol

Diabetes Visit	My Results	My Target
Date:		
Date:		
Date:		
Date:		

The American Diabetes Association LDL cholesterol target is below 100.

- **HDL cholesterol** is sometimes called the good cholesterol. It removes fat from your blood and keeps your blood vessels from getting blocked. Keeping HDL cholesterol **high** helps protect you from heart attack or stroke.

  The American Diabetes Association target for HDL cholesterol is different for men and women. The HDL cholesterol target for men is above 40. The HDL cholesterol target for women is above 50. Your diabetes health care team may set a different HDL target for you. Keep track of your results by using the chart below.

HDL Cholesterol

Diabetes Visit	My Results	My Target
Date:		
Date:		
Date:		
Date:		

The American Diabetes Association HDL cholesterol target is above 50 for women and above 40 for men.

- **Triglycerides** are another kind of blood fat that is linked to high blood sugar. High triglycerides raise your risk of a heart attack or stroke. Keeping your triglycerides **low** protects you.

   The American Diabetes Association target for triglycerides is below 150. Your diabetes health care team may set a different triglyceride target for you. Keep track of your results by using the chart below.

Triglycerides

Diabetes Visit	My Results	My Target
Date:		
Date:		
Date:		
Date:		

The American Diabetes Association triglycerides target is below 150.

   Bill's A-1-C, blood pressure, and cholesterol levels had been running high. He knew he needed to work on taking care of his diabetes ABCs. But it was hard to find time with the crazy hours of his retail job and having time for his family.

   He was grilling for a big family party when he had a sharp pain in his chest and felt short of breath. Bill told his wife, Denise, that he didn't feel right. Denise immediately called 911 to get Bill to the emergency room.

   Bill said, "They told me it was a heart attack. I'm feeling fine now, and I'm taking time to take care of my diabetes and my ABCs.

"I also found out that signs of a heart attack can be different for people with diabetes. Feeling sick to your stomach or short of breath, even without chest pain, is more common during a heart attack in people with diabetes."

What Are the Warning Signs of a Heart Attack?

- Chest pain or discomfort
- Pain or discomfort in your arms, back, jaw, neck, or stomach
- Shortness of breath
- Sweating or light-headedness
- Indigestion or nausea
- Tiredness

If you have warning signs of a heart attack, call 911. Doctors can take steps within an hour of the first warning signs of a heart attack to prevent further damage to your heart.

Robert woke up feeling very dizzy. He was so dizzy he couldn't get out of bed. He called his son to come over. Robert's son tried to help his dad to the bathroom, but Robert was having trouble walking. Robert's son decided to call 911. He thought his dad might be having a stroke.

Tests confirmed that Robert had had a mild stroke. He was treated right away. Now he's back home and doing well.

What Are the Warning Signs of a Stroke?

- Weakness or numbness on one side of your body
- Sudden confusion or trouble understanding
- Trouble talking
- Dizziness, loss of balance, or trouble walking
- Trouble seeing out of one or both eyes
- Double vision
- Severe headache

If you have one or more of these warning signs, call 911 right away. Getting treatment within hours can help prevent further damage to your brain.

Here's what Bill and Robert are doing to get their ABCs in their target range. Check the actions you want to do to take care of your diabetes ABCs:

1. **Change the way you eat by making wise food choices:**

   - Cut saturated fat in recipes.
   - Bake, broil, grill, or roast rather than frying.
   - Use cooking sprays and nonstick pans.
   - Choose lean meats and meat substitutes.
   - Take the skin off poultry.
   - Buy fat-free or low-fat dairy products, such as skim or 1% milk and low-fat cheeses.
   - Eat less fat that raises the risk of heart attack or stroke:

- **Saturated fat** is hard at room temperature. Butter, high-fat dairy products, and fatty meats all contain saturated fat.
- **Trans fat** is found in hydrogenated oils, margarines, and shortening. Trans fats are also found in baked products, such as cookies and crackers. Check the list of ingredients on food labels for hydrogenated fats.

- Eat fewer high-cholesterol foods, such as egg yolks, organ meats, high-fat meats, and dairy products.
- Two times a week, eat fish that contain fat that protects your heart. Examples are salmon, sardines, rainbow trout, herring, and mackerel.
- Choose good fats because they help lower cholesterol, such as canola oil or olive oil. Nuts also contain good fats.

Put a check mark next to the items above you'd like to try.

2. **Start a new exercise plan:**

- Think about an exercise routine you may want to start.
- Talk with your health care team about it and what's safe for you.
- Make a plan for when and where you'll get your exercise. See Chapter 10 for more about making a plan to get up and get going.

3. **Take medicines to lower blood pressure, blood sugar, and blood cholesterol, if you need them:**

- Many medicines can help you reach your ABC targets and lower your risk for a heart attack or stroke.
- Some types of blood pressure and cholesterol medicines can protect your heart. Talk with your doctor about which of these medicines are best for you.
- Aspirin can lower your risk of heart disease. Ask your provider if taking aspirin each day is right for you.

People with diabetes are at high risk for a heart attack, stroke, or PAD. Keeping your diabetes ABC numbers close to your targets helps reduce your risk. Talk with your health care team about what you can and will do to protect your heart and reduce your risk.

If you have warning signs of a heart attack or a stroke, call 911. If doctors can see you very soon after the first warning signs, they can prevent further damage.

Review warning signs with your family and friends. Tell them about calling 911 to get care right away.

Kidneys

Our kidneys filter our blood. They remove things that can harm us and keep things we need. People with diabetes can have kidney problems. This is also called nephropathy (neh-FROP-uh-thee).

When people have had diabetes for a long time, their kidneys may become damaged. High blood sugar and high blood pressure over time cause damage to the small blood vessels in the kidneys and reduce blood flow.

At Mama's last diabetes visit, her doctor checked her microalbumin. This is a urine test usually done once a year to check for small amounts of protein. Protein is not normally found in the urine. The results tell you how well your kidneys are working.

Mama's microalbumin was slightly elevated. Her doctor changed Mama's blood pressure medicine to an ACE inhibitor. Blood pressure medicines such as ACE inhibitors or ARBs protect your kidneys.

Mama also decided to work harder on lowering her blood sugar to get her A-1-C to her target. Any lowering of the A-1-C reduces the risk of diabetes problems, including kidney disease.

Early on, there might not be any warning signs of kidney problems. The kidneys work harder to make up for the damage. Later on, the kidneys may become worse. They may not be able to make up for the damage anymore. People may feel very tired or sick to their stomach. Their feet and hands may swell. Their skin may feel itchy. If kidney disease isn't found and treated, the kidneys will not be able to clean your blood. This is called kidney failure.

With kidney failure, dialysis will be needed to filter the blood. A kidney transplant is also an option.

The good news is that you can take steps to lower your risk for kidney problems.

- Have a microalbumin test every year. This is how you can find out early on if you have kidney damage and get treatment. Ask your doctor for your microalbumin results and record them in the following chart.

Microalbumin

Diabetes Visit	My Results
Date:	
Date:	
Date:	
Date:	

- Keep your blood sugar and A-1-C in your target range.
- Keep your blood pressure on target.
- Talk with your doctor about taking an ACE inhibitor or ARB.

Nerves

Diabetes can sometimes cause nerve damage. This is also called neuropathy (ne-ROP-uh-thee). The nerves in the feet and legs are the ones most often damaged. Sometimes the nerves in the hands and arms can also be affected.

Nerves that control the stomach, bladder, and digestion can sometimes be damaged. Also, nerve damage causes some people to have problems with having sex. For more on sex and diabetes, see Chapter 17.

When nerves become damaged by diabetes, some people **feel less** than before. Damaged nerves may not feel pain, heat, or cold.

Robert had lost feeling in his feet. He was out hiking with his buddies. He didn't notice the small stone that had gotten into his shoe. When he got home, he had a bad sore from that little stone he had walked on all day.

If the nerves in your feet are damaged like Robert's, you can't feel pain or an injury. Then a small injury can get worse and become a big problem.

When nerves become damaged by diabetes, some people **feel more** than before. If you feel less or if you feel more depends on what nerves are affected and how they are affected. You may feel burning or tingling. Aunt Carla complained about the weight of the sheets on her feet at night. She also had shooting pain in her legs and feet.

Denise was having low blood sugar a lot, even after eating all of her carbs at lunch or dinner. We checked her food records and logbook and saw patterns of low blood sugar. Her doctor did some tests and found that Denise had nerve damage that was affecting her stomach. She had gastroparesis (gas-TRO-puh-ree-sis). Gastroparesis happens when the nerves to the stomach are damaged or stop working. The stomach takes too long to empty. That's why Denise was having low blood sugars, even after eating her meals. Denise's doctor started her on medicine that helped. We also made changes in her meal plan.

The good news is that there are things you can do to protect yourself from nerve problems.

- Ask your health care provider to check your feet at least once a year to be sure your nerves are still sensitive.

- Check your feet every day for injuries, blisters, redness, or sores.
- Keep your blood sugar and A-1-C numbers in your target range.
- Talk with your health care team if you have any signs of nerve problems. There may be medicines or treatments that can help.

Chapter 20

What It All Means

Living with diabetes is hard. Learning to live with diabetes takes time and effort. Many of the things we do every single day affect our diabetes and blood sugar levels. The food we eat, how active we are, and how we handle stress all affect our diabetes. The choices you make on a daily basis affect your diabetes and your long-term risk for diabetes problems.

It takes time to take care of your diabetes. Some things may be easier for you, and some things may be harder. For someone else, it may be the other way around.

As you learn more about diabetes and about yourself, you'll learn ways that are easier for you to take care of your diabetes. Make the easier changes first. Take one step at a time.

Learn to lean on your family, friends, and diabetes health care team when you need help and support. Tell them what you need. Is it someone to talk to? Is it someone to walk with? Is it someone to share your problems with? Is it someone to help with shopping? Is it someone to start dinner? Is it someone to cook a healthy meal for you once a week? Is it someone to help with your medicines?

Many people I work with feel guilty a lot. They feel guilty about their diabetes care. They blame themselves when things aren't going right. When their blood sugar levels aren't in their target range, they think it must be their fault. They've done something wrong or they haven't done something they should have done. The truth is that sometimes we just don't know why a person's blood sugar is high. Do the best you can each and every day and let it go.

When you're feeling guilty, think about what could be going on. Are you stressed out? Do you need a change in your diabetes meal plan? Do you need diabetes medicine or a change in your medicine? So many factors affect your diabetes and your diabetes ABCs.

Don't feel guilty or blame yourself for being out of your target range. Seek the help and support you need from your diabetes team—your health care team and your family and friends. If you don't think your health care providers are right for you, think about going to other diabetes providers. After all, if you don't like your hairdresser, you go to someone else.

Remember to reward yourself for making changes and making progress. A reward can be as simple as taking the time to do something you enjoy. It can be time to read the newspaper, to watch a movie, to go to the park, to visit a garden, to take a hot bath, or to listen to music. Rewards can also be small purchases. You can buy yourself a flower, a magazine, or a CD. A long-term reward could be a weekend trip or a new pair of shoes.

I'll end this book with the way I started it. When it comes to your diabetes care, you are in charge. You choose what and how much to eat. You decide if you'll take your medicines, if you'll check your blood sugar, and if you'll be active. You decide to make and keep your office visits with your health care team.

By taking these actions to care for your diabetes, you'll feel better and have more energy. You can have your share of the good news that long-term diabetes problems can be delayed or even prevented. And taking care of your diabetes can also help to slow or reverse long-term diabetes problems that may have already started.

Take the first step toward your healthier life today!

Chapter 21

Diabetes Tools

This section contains tools that may be helpful to you in taking care of your diabetes:

- A list of carbohydrate foods you can use with carb counting
- A log to keep track of your blood sugars
- A chart for listing your medicines
- A calendar for meal planning
- A shopping list

Carbohydrate Serving Sizes

The number of carb servings that is right for you depends on your weight, age, and how active you are. A carb serving is about 15 grams of carbohydrate. Eating three or four carb servings at each meal and one or two carb servings for snacks works well for many people. By checking your blood sugar, you'll find out if your meal plan is working for you or if it needs to be tweaked.

You and your dietitian can make a meal plan that fits you. It needs to take into account your likes, dislikes, schedule, and diabetes target goals. Most people need their meal plans reviewed and revised once a year. Look on this as your 25,000-mile checkup.

The amount of carbs you eat affects your blood sugar more than anything else you eat, such as protein or fats. The list below shows the size of one carb serving.

Each carb serving below contains about 15 grams of carbohydrate:

Starches

1/4 bakery bagel
1 slice bread
1/2 English muffin, hot dog bun, or hamburger bun
1 small pita
3/4 cup ready-to-eat cereal
1/2 cup cooked cereal
1 6-inch tortilla
1 waffle or pancake the size of a CD, 1/4 inch thick
6–8 crackers

1/3 cup pasta or rice (brown or white)
1/2 cup beans, corn, peas, mashed or boiled potato, sweet potato, or winter squash
A handful (about 3/4 ounce) baked chips, pretzels, or low-fat snack crackers
3 cups light microwave popcorn

Fruits

1 small fresh fruit (about 4 ounces)
1/2 cup unsweetened canned fruit
1/4 cup dried fruit

2 tablespoons raisins
15–17 grapes
1/2 cup fruit juice
1 cup melon
1 cup berries

Milk

1 cup fat-free or low-fat milk
1 small carton plain or flavored yogurt (up to 100 calories)
1 cup fat-free or low-fat soy or rice milk

Sweets and Desserts

1 2-inch square cake or brownie, unfrosted

2 small cookies (2–3 ounces)

1/2 cup ice cream or frozen yogurt

1/4 cup sherbet or sorbet

Combo Foods

These foods mix carbohydrates with protein and fats. They contain different amounts of carbohydrate:

1 cup casserole or chili—2 carb choices and 2 meat servings

2 cups chow mein and 1 cup rice—3 carb choices and 2 meat servings

1 beef burrito—3 carb choices, 1 meat serving, and 2 fat servings

1/4 of a 10-inch cheese pizza with thin crust—2 carb choices, 2 meat servings, and 2 fat servings

1 medium serving fast-food French fries—4 carb choice and 4 fats

Free Foods

These foods contain a small amount of carbohydrate and less than 20 calories per serving. You can usually eat as much as you want, but if a serving size is given, limit the food to three servings per day to keep your blood sugar in your target range:

1 tablespoon catsup

1 tablespoon fat-free cream cheese, mayonnaise, or salad dressing

Sugar-free Jell-O

Lemon juice

Mustard

Nonfat cooking spray

1/4 cup salsa

Diet soft drinks

Spices and herbs

My Blood Sugar Log

Date	Time	Breakfast	Medicine/Comments	Time	Lunch	Medicine/Comments	Time	Dinner	Medicine/Comments	Time	Snack/Other	Medicine/Comments

Source: From the Diabetes and Cardiovascular Disease Toolkit, Blood Glucose Log, Kit #26.

My Medicines

Name and Strength* of Medicine	Used for	How Much to Take	When to Take	Notes**	Date Started
Over-the-counter, medicines, vitamins, herbs, home remedies					

*Strength means the number of milligrams (mg) or other units. You can find this information on the label.
**Foods or other medicines that should not be taken with this medicine, side effects, and other notes.
Source: From the Diabetes and Cardiovascular Disease Toolkit, Managing Your Medicines, #24.

My Meal Plans

Week of _____

	Sunday	Monday	Tuesday
Breakfast			
Snack			
Lunch			
Snack			
Dinner			
Snack			
	Activity Today	**Activity Today**	**Activity Today**

My Meal Plans *continued*

Wednesday	Thursday	Friday	Saturday
Activity Today	**Activity Today**	**Activity Today**	**Activity Today**

My Shopping List

Vegetables

Canned, Fresh, Frozen, In Season

☐ Asparagus
☐ Broccoli
☐ Carrots
☐ Eggplant
☐ Garlic
☐ Greens: collards, turnip
☐ Lettuce
☐ Onions
☐ Peppers: red or green
☐ Potatoes: new or baking
☐ Spinach
☐ Sweet potatoes
☐ Tomatoes
☐ _____
☐ _____

Fruit

Canned, Fresh, Frozen, In Season

☐ Apples
☐ Bananas
☐ Blueberries
☐ Cantaloupes
☐ Grapes
☐ Kiwi
☐ Lemons, limes
☐ Oranges
☐ Pears
☐ Raspberries
☐ Strawberries
☐ _____
☐ _____

Whole-Grain Products

☐ Bagels
☐ Bread, whole wheat
☐ Cereals: ready-to-eat, hot
☐ Crackers: low-fat
☐ English muffins
☐ Flour
☐ Pasta
☐ Rice: brown, converted white
☐ Rolls
☐ Tortillas: corn, whole wheat
☐ _____
☐ _____

Meat, Poultry, Fish

Canned, Fresh, Frozen

☐ Beef: loin, round, sirloin
☐ Chicken
☐ Deli meats: turkey, ham
☐ Fish
☐ Pork: chops, loin, tenderloin
☐ Shellfish
☐ Tuna fish: water-packed
☐ Turkey
☐ _____
☐ _____

Dairy Products

☐ Butter
☐ Cheese: low-fat
☐ Cottage cheese: low-fat
☐ Egg or egg substitutes
☐ Margarine: trans-fat free
☐ Milk: skim, 1%
☐ Yogurt: plain, light
☐ _____
☐ _____

Packaged Foods

☐ Beans: canned or dried, black, navy, pinto
☐ Frozen dinners: low-fat
☐ Pasta sauces
☐ Soups
☐ Tomato: paste, sauce
☐ _____
☐ _____

Snacks and Desserts

☐ Chips: baked potato, tortilla
☐ Cookies: low-fat, wafers, fruit-filled
☐ Dried fruit: apples, prunes, raisins
☐ Jell-O/pudding: sugar-free
☐ Ice cream, frozen yogurt: low-fat, sugar-free
☐ Jam, jelly: sugar-free
☐ Nuts
☐ Popcorn: low-fat
☐ Pretzels
☐ Whipped topping: low-fat
☐ _____
☐ _____

Drinks

☐ Coffee, tea
☐ Drinks, drink mixes: sugar-free
☐ Juices, light cranberry, orange, tomato, veggie
☐ _____
☐ _____

Condiments

☐ Catsup
☐ Honey
☐ Mayonnaise: low-fat
☐ Mustard
☐ Olives: green, black
☐ Pepper
☐ Pickles: low-salt, sugar-free
☐ Salad dressing: low-fat
☐ Salsa
☐ Seeds: sesame, pumpkin, sunflower
☐ Salt
☐ Spices, herbs
☐ Sugar, sugar substitutes
☐ Syrup: sugar-free
☐ Vinegars: balsamic, cider, red wine, rice wine, white wine
☐ _____
☐ _____

Other Items

☐ Baking powder
☐ Baking soda
☐ Cooking oils: canola, olive
☐ Cooking sprays
☐ _____
☐ _____

Pharmacy

☐ Blood pressure medicines
☐ Cholesterol medicines
☐ Diabetes medicines
☐ Strips for checking blood sugar
☐ Other prescription medicines
☐ Over-the-counter medicines
☐ _____
☐ _____

Index

About the American Diabetes Association

The American Diabetes Association is the nation's leading voluntary health organization supporting diabetes research, information, and advocacy. Its mission is to prevent and cure diabetes and to improve the lives of all people affected by diabetes. The American Diabetes Association is the leading publisher of comprehensive diabetes information. Its huge library of practical and authoritative books for people with diabetes covers every aspect of self-care—cooking and nutrition, fitness, weight control, medications, complications, emotional issues, and general self-care.

To order American Diabetes Association books: Call 1-800-232-6733. Or log on to http://store.diabetes.org

To join the American Diabetes Association: Call 1-800-806-7801. www.diabetes.org/membership

For more information about diabetes or ADA programs and services: Call 1-800-342-2383. E-mail: AskADA@diabetes.org or log on to www.diabetes.org

To locate an ADA/NCQA Recognized Provider of quality diabetes care in your area: www.ncqa.org/dprp

To find an ADA Recognized Education Program in your area: Call 1-888-232-0822. www.diabetes.org/recognition/education.asp

To join the fight to increase funding for diabetes research, end discrimination, and improve insurance coverage: Call 1-800-342-2383. www.diabetes.org/advocacy

To find out how you can get involved with the programs in your community: Call 1-800-342-2383. See below for program Web addresses.

- *American Diabetes Month:* educational activities aimed at those diagnosed with diabetes—month of November. www.diabetes.org/ADM
- *American Diabetes Alert:* annual public awareness campaign to find the undiagnosed—held the fourth Tuesday in March. www.diabetes.org/alert
- *The Diabetes Assistance & Resources Program (DAR):* diabetes awareness program targeted to the Latino community. www.diabetes.org/DAR
- *African American Program:* diabetes awareness program targeted to the African American community. www.diabetes.org/africanamerican
- *Awakening the Spirit: Pathways to Diabetes Prevention & Control:* diabetes awareness program targeted to the Native American community. www.diabetes.org/awakening

To find out about an important research project regarding type 2 diabetes: www.diabetes.org/ada/research.asp

To obtain information on making a planned gift or charitable bequest: Call 1-888-700-7029. www.diabetes.org/ada/plan.asp

To make a donation or memorial contribution: Call 1-800-342-2383. www.diabetes.org/ada/cont.asp